Muzungu Wendy

a woman's crusade against AIDS

Wendy Arnold, MPH

Dedication

This book is dedicated to my friends with HIV/AIDS who courageously contributed love and inspiration to my international challenges. I also thank my family for their endless support and encouragement throughout the years of HIV/AIDS trainings and adventures. They have taught me the real meanings of humility and passion.

Table of Contents

A New Year's Eve

It was about 8:30 p.m., and I was sitting in a posh restaurant at a half-empty circular table set for six near a wall of clear glass overlooking the Marina del Rey harbor, waiting for midnight. The only person I knew was the woman who had invited me here. Bette was a writer and we had been planning to jointly produce a TV series.

Bette had flown in from Colorado with a woman friend for this party and had managed to wangle an invitation for me too. Although I've never liked going to parties where I know no one, I decided to follow my own advice to check out anything or anyone unexpectedly crossing my path. Maybe we'd meet someone who could help launch our series. This was Los Angeles, after all.

So the three of us were picking at shrimp cocktails, and it was clear we'd come too early, since few other guests had arrived. Our host also noticed this and came over to speak with us, asking what we did for a living. After a few

1

minutes he excused himself. As we resumed our nibbling and empty chatter, our host suddenly reappeared with a woman in tow, emphatically stating that this was someone we had to meet, then rushed off again.

The lady—Wendy Arnold, slim, blond, looking to be in her late forties—turned out to be an AIDS educator. I started to question her about her work, and she began telling us of teaching about HIV/AIDS in Africa. Africa? She pushed ahead. This woman had enough energy to light up all of West L.A.! Stories about her work poured out of her in a cascade. They were fascinating, touching, shocking, and tragic.

As a writer and director, I know a good tale when I hear one. "You need to write a book," I interrupted.

"Everyone tells me that," said the blond Wendy, "but I can't write."

I don't know what came over me, because I answered, "I'll help you." Did I really say that? To a woman I'd met only ten minutes ago? Well, that's the effect Wendy has on people.

I told her I'd mail her a copy of my first book, The Search For David, *and if she liked my writing, we could talk further. She gave me her address, then shot off to somewhere else in the room. I didn't see her again that evening.*

But, as Rick said in the film Casablanca, *"This is the beginning of a beautiful friendship."*

And, yes, Wendy has lit up West L.A.—and a lot of Africa, not to mention parts of Europe, Russia, Israel, and—well, this is her story, it's important, it's gripping, it's brutally real, and you need to read it.

George Schwimmer, Ph.D.

Introduction

For many, many years, people have asked me when I would write a book, when would I share my experiences about my life, PEP/LA and PEP/International. What about my experiences on the streets of Los Angeles or in the alleys of neighboring Venice, where I was knifed by a young man? Or walking through communities of Uganda and hearing young kids scream at me, "Muzungu, Muzungu!"? Or picking up injured people by the side of the road and becoming best friends with them?

For years, people have been asking when I would share the anguish and the despair and the happiness and brilliant snapshots of life that are embedded in my memory. People have been saying, "Why do you keep doing what you do, where does your drive come from, what keeps you motivated, how do you stay committed, where does all your compassion come from?"

People have been envious because I love my work. I

love the diversity of each and every day, whether it's talking with homeless and runaway youth at Children of the Night or visiting a transition house for drug addicts or walking through the muck and mire of Skid Row, then changing clothes to give a presentation at a Catholic high school.

I want to share these experiences, and I'm not much of a writer, though God knows, I can talk! I want to share to let people know that one person *can* make a difference. I never thought that I really would make a difference because during high school I was told that I was an under-achiever, more of a trouble-maker and only an average B student. They thought I was indifferent to academics, so I was told to major in physical education and focus more on sports.

I guess I've mystified them because one person *can* make a difference.

I made a choice to get to the front lines and have the hands-on experiences, and it's a decision that's benefited me a great deal because it's given me different perspectives of what I *do* have, more than what I *don't* have, and has helped me understand that although I have many challenges due to osteo-arthritis, this is *nothing* compared to the debilitating emotional, psychological and physiological problems that my friends with AIDS have.

I am writing this book to show an appreciation for the experiences so that others understand that it's OK to break from conformity. I want you to take this journey with me, a journey that is sporadic, a journey that takes us through the United States and through many other countries around the globe. A journey that I hope has made me a better person.

I have an intense commitment to fight the HIV/AIDS epidemic and provide care, compassion and hope for people living with HIV disease. I have a lot of anger about this situation. I have a lot of frustration that people continue to die because they do not have the needed information, that people die because there is an anathema on the subject of sex. These are people who die from ignorance, and many of them are good people. It makes me angry that I discuss the same issues year after year after year, letting youth know that an HIV infection is avoidable. I have been saying the same thing now for thirty-two years.

When I started my work in 1982 there were 593 registered AIDS cases and now in 2014 there are more than 1.4 million. What is wrong? Why do the numbers continue to escalate out of control? I have to take this anger and frustration and put it into something productive.

My way of getting back at the virus is by giving people information, 'fighting the fears with the facts'. This is a *disease*, not a disgrace. There are a lot of diseases in the world. Why is there such a stigma and discrimination about AIDS?

I am also writing this book to normalize the discussion of sensitive subjects, such as sexuality. Sexual activity is a normal biological process. If we can't talk about it, it will be driven underground and be more irresponsible. It will be the forbidden fruit, and then everybody will want to try it. But if we *can* talk about sex respectfully, nonjudgmentally and honestly and present the choices that can be made, then we *can* begin to deal with the health issues associated with sexual activity.

I also owe it to my family to write this book because they have been so supportive.

And to George Schwimmer, Ph.D., who met with me weekly on Wednesday mornings, week after week, with his tape recorder in hand, as he patiently listened to my diatribe of stories and emotions, then went with me to three or four sessions, contributed two chapters and helped me to shape much of this book.

Then there is Africa. There is so much desperation, poverty and wrong information. The myths obscure the facts: In Zimbabwe, 1999, I was told that A.I.D.S. is the acronym for the **A**merican **I**nvention to **D**iscourage **S**ex, not the Acquired Immune Deficiency Syndrome. Yet there is a special receptivity, there is an insatiable thirst and hunger for what I tell them.

The epidemic is absolutely devastating with estimations that each day more than 9,000 are infected with HIV, 7,000 dying from AIDS-related complications. And nobody really knows the accurate numbers because people are not getting tested, and many Africans are dying from common diseases like malaria, TB and pneumonia—

diseases also associated with HIV/AIDS.

I have met many Africans who initially feel helpless and hopeless, yet when they see an enthusiastic white girl, a "Muzungu," it's a beacon of hope and importance. They share their lives, traditions and precious values—they are genuine and hospitable. A smile is universal.

I love Africa.

Choices

What do I want to do in my work? To motivate, to empower more people to and share the emotions that go with them.

I want to be an inspiration for others: "I did this, so you can do it, too. I want you to do it." To stand up for their own will, and for them to be strong. I want people to say, "That girl from Concord, Massachusetts—if she can do it, I can do it."

I will never tell anyone what to do. I want a person to make the choice and then feel good about it. I cannot say, "You *should* take the HIV antibody test." I want to discuss the advantages, the disadvantages. "*You* can make the decision," because ultimately we all make decisions. And we screw up a lot. I sure have screwed up, and that's one of the reasons I openly give my training materials, evaluations and surveys to people—what's the point of someone starting from point 'A' again? I've *done* that, I've *made* all these mistakes, so why should they repeat them? And time is running out. People are dying.

I'll drop everything to help someone. People call and say, "You're the first live voice—you're the first person who hasn't put me on hold—who's willing to talk with me, who's willing to follow up and who's shown any compassion for my needs." When the tone is urgent, you can't say you'll call them back tomorrow. I take the call immediately, clear away the desk so I can really concentrate on the issue.

One evening, I talked with a girl for three hours. Why? Because she needed to talk. She was scared of her husband and the police were there as she cried out, "I want my Mommy, I want my Mommy!" She has neurological problems and has trouble understanding even the most basic facts. I know she's desperately alone and I know I'm her only friend. I was the maid of honor at her wedding. I was exhausted after talking with her, but it was a good exhaustion.

I'm also very stubborn. I don't put up with bullshit

anymore. I sometimes shoot from the hip and then realize, "Ooh, I shouldn't have said that." But there are times when somebody really ticks me off, especially when it's a homophobic comment.

There was one time I was playing tennis at Plummer Park in West Hollywood with a gay friend—I mean everything I do is with gay guys—what's the big deal, it's a non-issue for me. I've been a surrogate member of the gay community for thirty-two years now!

Anyway, these two rough-looking Russian guys came up to me and whined, "Hey, pretty lady, why are you playing with a faggot?" I didn't appreciate that comment. I put down my tennis racket and went over to him—I didn't even *think*—and said, "Excuse me, what did you say?"

"Why're you playing with the fag? He's a fag – you're playing with a fag, aren't you?"

I said, "He's my *friend*, and I *don't* see any need for that kind of language." Then he *pushed* me a little bit, I pushed him *back*, he hauled off and slapped me, flattened me, and sang out, "Fag hag, fag hag." Then both of them took off laughing.

So I'm not very good about keeping my mouth shut when I should. But you know what? It's OK to step outside of the 'sacred circle,' it's OK to get slapped around a bit, because the *benefits* and the satisfaction far outweigh the emotional regret of having done nothing. I also *choose* to get involved, instead of just passing by.

One evening in Cameroon, about eight in the evening, we were driving to a dinner with colleagues, a bush meet, and on the way we saw tufts of grass on the road ahead of us. When there is an accident, people pull up big tufts of dirt and plants and put them on the roadway to slow the oncoming traffic. It's like the flares we use in the U.S. Really quite clever. We could see all the bunches of plants and knew something had happened.

As we got closer, we could see that in the middle of the road there was the crumpled body of a woman who had been hit by a car. I asked our driver to pull over to the side. I just wanted to see if there was anything we could do for her. I don't know *why* I even thought it was our business, but he stopped the car and I ran over to the woman.

There were people all around her and all I could hear

them mumbling to each other was that she was "a mad woman," so it was her fault. "She is 'a mad woman,' and mad women deserve to get hit." People say that so they will not be liable for what happened or they will not be responsible for her death.

The woman lay lifeless in the road, but I could see that she *wasn't* "a mad woman." She was a well dressed young pregnant woman carrying a basket of what had probably been nicely arranged leafy vegetables. I immediately felt for her carotid pulse. Nothing, absolutely nothing. Then I felt for a pulse on the other side of her head and there was nothing there either. When my eyes adjusted to the darkness of night I could look closer at her. I felt the wetness of her brain at my fingers and saw that the entire top of her skull had been ripped off by the accident.

Some of the Cameroonians speak English, some French, and mostly they speak 'pidgin', a combination of several dialects. I could hear broken phrases of English, so I whispered, "Could we please pray for this woman?" I don't remember the words that I blurted out, and there were two others who then spoke. When I got back into the car I was careful not to touch anyone or anything because I had blood all over me. An hour later, when we got to the bush meet, I quietly washed the blood off.

After the dinner meeting, on the way back to the Baptist Convention Center in Mutengene, where four of us shared a room, I noticed that her body was still there, now on the side of the road. It really bothered me—the disrespect, the indignity, the lack of concern. Why was this young woman just *left* there, abandoned like an animal carcass? I felt sick. The next morning, at seven o'clock, we traveled the same road, and I was horrified to see she was still there. I said, "Please stop the car." I was wearing a little petticoat underneath my long skirt and I took it off and covered her, for her own privacy and for her transition to another world.

That situation significantly wounded me. I don't know why I stopped and I don't know why it concerned me so much. But I impulsively *do* things like that.

Another time in Limbe, Cameroon, I was discussing medical treatments at the Doctor's Hospital when I heard the frantic "honk, honk, honk" from a taxi roaring toward the entrance. Should I get involved? My response was instinctual as I ran to the car. There was a woman in the back seat *covered* with blood, *covered* with blood. She'd been in an accident.

She continued to moan as people ran around chaotically. Often they peered in the window to get a better view and just stared. I stood motionless waiting for a cue to move. The nurses continued to circle the car with disorganized gasps for about fifteen minutes, and no one was *doing* anything about the woman in the car. They were just looking at her, and I finally exclaimed to one of my doctor friends, "That woman needs help!"

Could I stop the bleeding, could I provide some emotional support? Without hesitation, I crawled in next to her, and she was just saying, "Oh, Jesus, oh, Jesus, oh Jesus, oh...." I could see that her whole left eye had been ripped out and she had a compound fracture of her left arm. The bones jutting out were terrifying. I held her right hand and tried to be reassuring with, "You're going to be O.K," and, "Yes, Jesus is with you." She was still crying, "Oh, Jesus, oh, Jesus."

There was still no medical assistance although several

hospital staff members were walking about in confusion. As she gazed at me I could see that she was calming down. Her voice was less urgent as she rocked back and forth. She told me her name was Margaret and that she had been in an accident with her sister. But where was her sister? Why wasn't anyone helping her?

Then one of the doctors cautioned me about my getting exposed to HIV from all the blood. That was it! They were afraid of HIV! That's why no one came to her assistance! But I did not feel in danger, as I quickly remembered that I had no open cuts. Finally, four nurses came and put Margaret on a canvas stretcher. They were visibly uncomfortable as they positioned her large and bloodied body.

The next day, for the second session of my workshop, I slipped away to hospital admissions to see if I could find Margaret. One of the nurses smiled and said, "She was hoping to see you." I went to her room where she had about five of her family members clustered by her bed. When they saw me, they said, "Oh, *you're* the white girl she was talking about. She thinks you saved her life. You're the white girl!"

I looked at our patient and said, "Hi, Margaret, it's good to see you are doing better." She looked up at me, started crying and said, "White girl—Wendy, white girl, you saved my life. You helped me to communicate with God."

And there was such a *rush* of feelings inside me....

Why I do these things, I don't know—I just get *involved.*

Like the motorcycle accident at Westwood and Olympic in West Los Angeles. This guy was going too fast in the right-hand lane and a car cut him off. I saw the bike scatter, as did he. I pulled over and jumped out to help him. I was hesitant about seeing how messed up he might be and was almost relieved to find that he only had an intense laceration on his left knee, but he was in severe pain and there was glass everywhere.

I slowed traffic down and then huddled beside him until the ambulance came. He was Russian and appreciated my broken sentences in Russian mannerisms. Other motorists stopped to retrieve pieces of the motorcycle from the pavement. Then I noticed that my knees were pretty badly cut up. I didn't even feel it.

I finally got back into my car and shook uncontrollably – I was in *shock*. I went home and immediately called my Mum, my best friend and source for reliable moral support. Of course this was not fair to her because what could she do from Boston when I was in California?

Why do I just *happen* to be in places at times like that? I don't know. But I *choose* to get involved, once there. That's what life is all about. Choices. Involvement.

Perspective

My experiences during the previous three weeks in Uganda had left me with deep feelings of despair, followed by hope, then with greater passion for my HIV/AIDS work. I was finally back in West Los Angeles, though, yearning for a swim to loosen jetlagged muscles. As I entered my L.A. sports club, whiffs of salmon, pasta and gourmet salads wafted out to me from the restaurant— quite different from the *mutumbo* made of goat intestine filled with goat stomach that was the staple food of Kayunga, Uganda and Chivende, Zimbabwe.

I watched club members carelessly discard half-eaten sandwiches that could feed at least four children for two days in Bukolooto, saw impeccably uniformed club attendants with spotless trays swoop down on the discards and whisk them off to large plastic waste containers. In India, garbage would lie exposed outside, covered in seconds with flies and vermin—only emaciated dogs would dare to pick through the piles of vomit, human feces, and animal entrails strewn on the ground. I pensively walked from the restaurant to the ladies locker room to change into my bathing suit.

At poolside, I dipped my left foot into the crystal clear water of the twenty-five-meter swimming pool. It was warm, like the Bagmati River in Nepal, though there were no cremation ashes from a Hindu funeral floating on the water.

"Hey, Wendy, where've you been," wafted a voice across the pool. It was a friend, Frank. He massaged his tanned pectorals and sucked in those perfectly chiseled abdominals as he waited for my answer.

In Cebu City, the Philippines, the ribs of begging orphans protruded through their chests, with no muscles— just stomachs bloated from starvation. Frank's stride as he came over to me was confident and strong, not like the women infected with HIV/AIDS in Kikamba, Kenya, who limped and crawled from the pain of neuropathy.

"I was back in Africa, Frank, doing HIV/AIDS prevention through peer education trainings."

22

A flood of memories surged through me—jubilant tribal dances, eating greasy *sadza* with friends, identifying Ugandan roommates in the dark only by their perfect white teeth when they smiled, meeting hundreds of AIDS orphans, and sharing tears with a woman who had just buried her son.

I shook off the images, returned to the present and asked, *"And how're you doing, Frank?"*

Frank took a ceremoniously deep breath and sighed, *"I've had absolutely the worst day today! The mechanic of my Mercedes is out of town and my cell phone has been getting terrible reception."*

He carefully rubbed oil onto his shaved legs to protect his skin, skin so different from that of a Nepalese street child covered with lesions, boils and open sores—or the nauseous smell rising from the rotting wounds of injecting drug users in Puerto Rico that still live vividly in my mind. I cautiously returned Frank's glance but didn't answer him, instead slipped quietly into the pool. My goggles filled with tears.

I sank under the surface of the enveloping warm water,

23

the only sound my breath through the snorkel. I felt so alive in my life, yet so wounded by Frank's priorities. The juxtaposition of the horrors I'd seen over the past twenty years and the opulence that Frank took for granted shook my sense of reality. Did he and I really live in the same world? Was he even aware of my world? How could he just wrap himself in his cocoon of expensive cars and cell phones?

Why was he on the path of material accumulation, while I was spending precious time begging for funds to finance my work? Why did I cherish taking risks with drug addicts, street children, orphans and countless people with HIV/AIDS? Where did my insatiability, to reach just one more person with the message of hope, come from? What gave Frank his psychological 'high,' when my 'high' was a smile, a thank you, a hug or just the feeling of acceptance in a tiny Kenyan village? Where did my drive come from? Why had I even chosen the field of HIV/AIDS education?

I began to swim, each stroke bringing another thought or question into my mind. It all comes down to choices, I realized. "Why" doesn't matter, only how I feel about what I chose. I feel good! I feel great! What a life I've led!

Michael

When Michael died, I…couldn't *feel* myself, I couldn't *breathe*, I didn't –

Michael was one of my very best friends.

He was from Boston and had come to Los Angeles in the early '90s with an AIDS diagnosis. I met him around 1995. Since I'd been reared around Boston, in Concord, Michael and I had a mutual respect and nostalgia for the east coast and our New England friends—how different they were from the melting-pot population of Los Angeles. That perspective opened the doors to our friendship.

Michael was a gentle man. Just being around him was calming. We could sit for hours without words and have total communication in that silence. If he took a deep breath and slowly exhaled, I'd look at him pensively, and say, "Penny for your thoughts, babe." He'd take another breath and respond "I was just thinking about how perfect that plant looks on my balcony. Look at those leaves reaching up to God and the unknown."

Michael had such serenity in spite of his AIDS.

I'd be so proud of him when he'd join a team of PEP/LA peer educators for talks with the teens about HIV/AIDS prevention. His contribution to the discussions always was to personify the epidemic with his testimony of having to live with the challenges of AIDS. He'd be so very calm as he explained how difficult it was to feel like 'a walking time bomb,' never knowing when the next disease or complication might be the end for him.

He'd say, "If I had heard about how to prevent HIV infection when I was your age, I wouldn't be going through this nightmare of uncertainty, loss of control and total dependence on medicines that make me so sick." Oftentimes there would be just a deafening silence of sadness as he encouraged the teens to keep themselves safe. He was so vulnerable and yet so courageous to stand before audiences and openly admit that he had AIDS.

When the complications of AIDS compromised Michael's independence, we set up a schedule of who would spend the night with him in his little apartment. I treasured those nights of 'spooning' and snuggles, but he never was able to sleep for more than a couple of minutes at a time because of all of the pain. He'd get up and pace, then reluctantly return to bed with yet another deep sigh.

There also were night sweats, when we'd strip his pajamas, towel him dry, change his sheets, and turn on his little fan. Then came chills, more night sweats, more frustration, and finally the stone silence of the unknown. Sometimes he would only get a couple of hours of rest before the sun came up. It always hurt me more to sense his pain than to experience any pain of my own. I felt helpless and hopeless and could only offer him soft words of encouragement.

But he got progressively sicker.

On November 17, 1998, I picked up a message from Michael's uncle. It was 10:30 p.m., and I was feeling pretty good after an hour of exercise and a toasty sauna. I usually don't check my home answering machine that late but something didn't feel right to me this evening. I pushed the message button. My heart sank when I heard the tone of Uncle Donald's first words, "Wendy, dear, Michael has taken a turn for the worse, and we don't think there is much time." I felt my heart pounding rapidly in my throat, and my legs were suddenly weak.

I lived in West Los Angeles, the hospital was in Tarzana—a thirty minute drive. I sped over the freeways, pushing the car to twenty miles above the speed limit. I didn't care if I got a ticket—I had to get there as fast as I could. I pulled into the first parking space I saw at the hospital, rushed to the front doors. I tried to look calm as I entered the lobby and went past some nurses. I knew that if you walk fast, they don't bother you.

When the elevator doors closed, I angrily punched '4.' I'm not sure where the anger came from. The fourth floor was oncology, since Michael, in addition to all his other illnesses, was riddled with cancer. When the elevator doors opened, I quickened my step. The nurses at their desks recognized me but showed no emotion. Now I was really worried. I pushed on to Michael's room.

Michael was in a coma, did respond to my voice and touch, although his eyes stared blankly. He was just skin and bones now, and for someone with so many high fevers, his body felt very cold. I curled up next to him and encouraged him to let go, to 'reach for the Light.' "It's OK to stop fighting, Michael, time to release the pain. Do you see the Light? Do you feel its warmth? It's OK to go."

The room was filled with a cacophony of noises— clicking monitors, hissing oxygen pump, surging blood pressure machine, the drip, drip, drip of the intravenous fluid—rubbing my nerves raw. Then his relentlessly deep breathing, very slow, very deliberate. A long inhale, shorter exhale—again, again, in and out, in and out. I counted the deep sighs as I massaged his bony arm with the circular barbed wire tattoo wound around it.

All that *deep* breathing...and then, suddenly— *total*...silence.

The machines were deafening now. I nudged him, whispering "Michael?" No response. I could feel the urgency rising in my voice, "Michael, Michael?" Then I gently shook his left shoulder and implored, "Michael, please wake up! Michael, please wake up!" There was no response.

I can't remember even breathing then. For a moment I didn't seem to know who I was or who *he* was or where I was. I was in total shock. There was just this…vacuum separating my body from reality, and the weight of the air crushing me down. I was stunned, couldn't move. Shock.

Then the doctor came in and said, "I'm sorry, Wendy, he's gone."

What does he mean, 'He's gone,' I thought. *Michael's still here, he's just sleeping. Wait, wait, he'll breathe again, and the nightmare will end.* But I knew it wouldn't.

I stayed with Michael for a long time, praying beside him. I asked God's angels to be gentle as they took him to the unknown. The room seemed to vibrate and the light intensified. Was he still with me? I just held him. My mind raced with the memories: the love, his friends, the Speakers' Bureau, his spirituality, his mom Kathleen. I was dizzy, I was calm, I was angry—yet relieved. I felt empty, and so insignificant.

Then chaos.

Attendants came in and placed Michael in a heavy

black plastic body bag. I watched as they zipped it up to his chin.

"*Wait!*" I implored, "I want to say goodbye."

I cupped his face – it was so cold, so bony, so terribly terribly thin – and kissed him on his left cheek, a kiss that would stay in my mind forever. With a glance at the doctor, I finally blurted out, "OK, he's yours."

But when they closed the last bit of the zipper – the *sound* of that zipper closing, it *just* – cut into me. I'll never forget that. It will stay with me until I die. Every zipper from a backpack or poster bag or suitcase – it was a reminder of my last moments with Michael.

I went through all the Kubler-Ross stages of death and dying after Michael's death:

First, *Shock* – with Michael's last gasp of breath I felt that he sucked oxygen from my own lungs. Was I breathing at all? Why couldn't I feel my feet or hands? Where was I, and what were all those mechanical sounds?

Then, *Denial* – "No! He's just sleeping. Let me wake him now because he needs to take a breath. There, I think I felt his fingers move. The doctor made a mistake. He's not 'gone,' he's just about to take a breath." Years after his death, I'd still reach for the telephone to share news and then remember he isn't here.

Next, *Anger* – When Michael died, I was angry at AIDS, at God, at the medical system. Why wasn't there education in the schools? Why are the teachers avoiding any discussions about HIV/AIDS? I was angry with who I was, what I *couldn't do*, why I was still alive and he had to die from ignorance and unavailable information. I was angry at everyone and no one. So, I tried to squelch my anger and frustration by throwing myself into my work, to reach as many people as possible with my message of HIV/AIDS prevention.

And, *Bargaining* – I negotiated with God for Michael's return. Maybe if I prayed more often, or went to church, or was nicer to people, then he'd come back? Several weeks after his memorial service, I challenged myself to swim the entire length of the Sports' Club pool underwater, with no snorkel. *If* I could make it to the other side, Michael's death would only have been a bad dream that would be cancelled when I woke up. I nearly drowned and then was angry all over again because I had failed.

Now, *Depression* – After the memorial service, the 'Celebration of Life' and the cleaning up of his apartment, I was so empty, so lonely, so tired. I felt helpless, hopeless and guilty that I was still alive. "Please leave me alone." "No, I don't want to have you come over and try to cheer me up." "Please don't *ever* tell me, 'He's in a better place.'" I hate it when people say that to me! If you don't know what to say to a person in bereavement, *don't say anything at all!*

Finally, *Acceptance* – When would I ever accept that Michael really was dead? How could I when I was still in denial and thought perhaps he'd just gone out of town. That was it! He was visiting his family in Minnesota and would return next week! Even when I opened the urn to see his ashes, I could not accept that it really was Michael. Perhaps only now, when I see pictures of his gravestone, can I accept that Michael is gone.

And then I'd go back to anger or denial or bargaining or depression, and it would start all over again, jumbled together with subsequent AIDS deaths and bereavements. I

33

had to quiet my anger with more HIV/AIDS prevention work, I had to reach more people, I had to keep fighting that devil of HIV/AIDS and help those who have to live with it.

I relive Michael's death every time I speak about the psychology intertwined with HIV/AIDS. That's his legacy, his gift to the world. The emotions I feel about him push me on—he's on the speaker's platform with me, every time I talk about him. He may be dead to the world, but he's alive to me, working with me, hand in hand.

But the grief cycle has engulfed me repeatedly during my life—being totally rocked by what I saw and how I felt when someone I knew died: shock, denial, anger, bargaining, depression, acceptance. So much of that has been in my experience, all the way back to 1982, when people didn't really know what AIDS *was*.

Back to when I met Steve.

Steve

My work in HIV/AIDS and with people living with the disease started early in 1982, when there were only 1,600 AIDS cases in the United States. At first the disease was called GRID ('Gay Related Immunodeficiency Disease'), then, in 1983, the virus was LAV (lymphadenopathy-associated virus), and in 1984 HTLV I (Human T-cell Leukemia-lymphoma Virus Type I).

Living right next door to me were two guys—Steve, a pediatrician in his early forties, and his partner, Dan, an artist and a college teacher. Steve and I had a mutual love and admiration for gardening, planting and roses. He always had the most beautiful roses, which were much nicer than mine. His roses got to be three feet high, with thick stalks, while mine were just flimsy floppy, but he always loved it when I'd come over to help him with his roses.

One time, in September 1982, I saw Steve out in his

garden. It was hot, and he was sweating profusely. I knew he wasn't feeling well. He had told me, as he'd told the rest of the neighborhood, that he had cancer. I went out to help and talk with him. As we were digging away and pulling out weeds, he looked over at me and said, "I know—because of your background in public health—that you'll understand what I'm going to tell you."

And I replied, "Oh, this sounds serious."

He got up and said, "Wendy, I've got something called 'gay cancer.' They don't know anything about it, and I'm really scared."

I'd read about this "mysterious disease," an epidemic that was apparently caused by a virus inflicting only gay men. "How could that be possible," I wondered. I'd never heard of a disease that singled out specific populations. Researchers did not even know how it was transmitted and feared that it could be airborne.

I stood up, gave him a hug and said, "That must really hard for you because no one knows much about this."

His eyes welled up with tears, and he replied, "You're

the first person who's hugged me for more than six months."

"Why?" I asked.

"Because everyone thinks I'm going to give 'it' to them, and they've all been treating me like a leper. My doctor won't even let me come within three feet of him—when I walk into his office, he already has his gloves on. If the doctors do any examinations, they've got masks, gowns, glasses, gloves."

I said, "Steve, I don't think you can get it just by being around people."

"Everyone thinks it is gotten by casual contact," he whispered, his eyes looking at the ground.

I was quick to add, "I haven't heard anything about it being in the air. If it were airborne, it would be a pandemic striking all populations, young, old, black, white. But now this disease seems localized in mostly the gay community."

Steve was hospitalized several times after that, since

the disease progressed rapidly. The disease AIDS had only been identified in '81, and from '81' to '85 people were gone within two years of diagnosis. Miraculously, Steve was still alive in '85. But there was atrocious discrimination among medical personnel for people with AIDS at that time.

One afternoon early that year I went to visit Steve at the UCLA hospital. I had been doing some educational work in HIV/AIDS by then, talking to high school students and diverse adult groups as a volunteer speaker with AIDS Project Los Angeles (APLA). A lot of the discussions were to allay the fears of transmission by casual contact. But I'll never forget walking down the corridor to Steve's room.

The room was at the very end of the corridor. Outside his door there was a big sign: "BIO-HAZARD," yellow strips, "Danger," "Place contaminated objects here," "Please wear gowns and masks before entering." There was a tray of dried food hastily covered with napkins at the other side of the door.

I knocked, walked in, and said, "Steve, they're adding more signs—this is getting a bit much."

And he said, "Wendy, they're not coming near me. All they do is probe me and poke me and take more blood samples. Every time they come in, it's those gowns and masks."

"What about your food? It's outside in the corridor."

And he said, "They won't bring it in."

"How are you eating?"

"Only when visitors come."

I brought his food in, but it was cold and ugly. I told him to wait a minute, went down to the cafeteria, got him some sandwiches and cookies, then sat on the side of his bed and tried to encourage him to eat. But he wasn't hungry.

I said, "This room is freezing!"

And his answer, still so vivid for me after all this time, was, "They won't come in to turn the heat up."

That did it. I got up, went to the nurses' station and said, "Look, your patient, Dr. Steve, in room 4121, what's going on here? Why aren't you giving him his food, why aren't you turning up his heat?"

And she said, "He's got a terribly contagious disease."

"That is no way to treat someone," I answered, "Can't you at least tell me how to get some heat in this room?"

So, finally, this man walked in to Steve's room, and it looked like he was ready for a lunar walk. Plastic mask, rubber gloves up his arms.

"You're wearing all this just to turn up the heat?" I asked.

I mean, I was in tears at that point. This must have been so humiliating for him. I could see that Steve was very hurt by this. The only people who were giving him any human touch were his family and very close friends.

It angered me, so I had to take that anger and turn it into something concrete. Because if I didn't focus the frustration into something purposeful and positive, then it would have been misdirected, and I would have started yelling at checkout clerks in supermarkets and honking at little old ladies on the streets. I had to take the anger, frustration and sadness and do something with it. So I accepted a job as the full-time Community Outreach Coordinator with AIDS Project Los Angeles.

In September of '85 my black lab 'Cheo' was dying, and I knew I had to put her to sleep. She was getting so old, seventeen, and it was time for me to let her go. We justified her destination to 'Rainbow Bridge', a lovely location somewhere between Heaven and earth. I knew Steve was dying, too, and I talked to him and said, "Well, maybe you can go to Heaven together," because Steve loved Cheo. So, I timed my awful decision of putting her to sleep to coincide with his death. Steve died in September. He went to Heaven with Cheo.

Later, his partner, Dan, also developed AIDS, and as he got progressively sicker and sicker, I got very close to his mother, Ruby, and her second husband, Ed—and I'm still very close to them. When a person is dying, everyone is involved —"What can I do, how can I help?" Then the person dies, and everyone disappears. It's kind of like, "OK, that's over with." And they just leave. Well, I didn't do that with Ruby and Ed. I kept in touch with her and I still talk with her regularly.

I have a picture of Dan, who was a very, very entertaining man. He was always funny and even had a sense of humor about his AIDS. I take his picture with me in my international work. I take several pictures of my friends who are living with or who have died from HIV/AIDS. During my trainings, I'll frequently put the pictures out on a table, and say, "Look at those pictures—look very closely. These are the faces of AIDS in America." And I'll tell stories about each one of them.

I never had a picture of Steve, though, until January of 2004, when I mentioned to Ruby that Steve was really the one who had started my drive, started my anger, taking my frustration and sadness into an energy to really compel me to get active in AIDS prevention. And she sent me a picture of Steve. So now, after nineteen years, I *finally* have a picture of Steve, taken in 1981, when he was still healthy. When I received it I was in tears. I told her, "Ruby, I just can't tell you how much this means to me." Because at last I had a picture of the man who had motivated my passion to work in HIV/AIDS.

Family and High School

I was born early on November 9, 1947, in Boston, Massachusetts, the second child, a troublemaker from the beginning. I was due November 20, but apparently I could hardly wait to get out, so I pushed forward the due date. Mum told me it was rather inconvenient, because she was having an evening party, all the guests had arrived, and then it was, "Oh no, the baby is on the way," so I messed up her plans.

With all due respect to Grammy Arnold, my paternal grandmother, I inherited, and hated for my entire life, the formal name of *Virginia* W. Arnold. I was saved by Mum's stepbrother Wendell, because my middle name, Wendy, was a lot more agreeable to me than Virginia.

The name 'Virginia' also haunted me whenever I had to take standardized tests requiring the first 6 letters of my name, shortened to V-I-R-G-I-N. My high school friends would taunt me singing, "Virgin for short, but not for long!" Cute.

I had a three-years-older sister, Dorrie, and a one-year-younger brother, David. I always felt that Dorrie was the favored daughter, being the firstborn. When David arrived, it was like, yippee, it's a guy. So here was the favored older sister, the second daughter—just kind of daughter number two—and then brother David, who was born with a little golden spoon in his mouth, just because he was a boy.

We moved to Lockport, New York when I was around two. All I really can recall about our big brick house was that it was always very, very cold. I also remember the trundling one day down a sidewalk with Mum and my little red wagon, when out of nowhere a boxer—in my eyes absolutely huge, growling, vicious—attacked me. Apparently I wasn't really hurt but was now terrified of dogs. That's when Mum and Dad got Pango, a black Lab. I've been hooked on Labs ever since and will never be without one, two or three of them.

The next year we moved to Nashoba Road, Concord, Massachusetts. Dad was employed by a company that manufactured plastic bags, the sticky ones that never opened properly and got gooey when it was hot. To me, Dad was a genius. He had an MBA from Harvard, and I knew that was very important. Mum was more than just my Mum, she was my best friend. She was always welcoming when the school bus dropped me off at 2:15 p.m., and I could hardly wait to tell her about my incredibly exciting day in school. She also made the best banana bread one could imagine.

I was a 'war baby', now more idiomatically, euphemistically, called a 'baby boomer', whatever that means. The description is still an enigma for me, but, regardless of the label, in our neighborhood there were lots of us 'boomers': the Gills, Haskins, Hortons, Springs, Malcolms, Willets, Motleys, Moultons, Vanderpools, Baldwins, and too many others to mention.

We did everything together, on bicycles, roller skates, skateboards and skis. I fondly remember the early evening games of 'kick the can' and 'cops and robbers.' It was good clean fun, no cigarettes, no booze, no drugs, no sex— quite different from today's youngsters. And we soon learned to identify our different it's-time-for-dinner-bells as we were called home for evening meals.

For me, good, clean fun included pranks. I loved to

push the limits. There was the thrill of getting into trouble, the thrill of spying on people. If someone was having a big party, Susie Horton and I would go and spy, looking in windows and climbing up trees to get a better view. And I just loved lighting fires. Bundling pine needles in the Pollard's yard and making little bonfires was very exciting. Mum tried to discourage my pyromania by making me ignite long matchsticks and I had to burn them all the way to the very end, where I'd invariably suffer a burn.

Lighting little fires progressed into firecrackers and cherry bombs: *kaboom* went the Berger's mailbox and the precious lilacs carefully planted by Mr. Hickey. I didn't kill anybody but easily could have. When the lit cherry bomb hit the cinders in the unfortunate recipient's fireplace, there was a dramatic explosion, propelling bits of wood and sparks into the living room. It was an absolute delight. Then the sirens, red flashing lights and search whistles added to the thrill. I could hear the cops calling to each other as I'd scurry up a tree.

I do remember getting pulled quite often into the Concord police station. It was probably for the exploded mailboxes or broken street lights. Or maybe it was because

46

of the snow balls that I'd frozen for an assault on speeding cars along Elm Street. I think I remember it so well because I must have been quite small and the reception area desk was so very high that I had to stand on my tippy-toes to see who was at the top. The people in blue uniforms tried to intimidate me, but I thought it was all hilarious and just loved the attention.

My brother David encouraged my delinquency with 'dirty-dog double dares.' He designed the task, Wendy got caught. At Woolworth's, he dared me to put two perky little turtles into my cheeks, but then I had to buy some candy at the register, so I had to talk. The little turtles' tails peeked through my lips and I was severely reprimanded. And how was I to know that those mirrors all over Woolworth's were actually see-through windows for security surveillance? But I would still do anything for my brother David. There was a thrill in taking risks, and that thrill is still with me today.

My sister Dorrie, being older and more mature, had different friends and didn't participate with our childish games. I got all her hand-me-down clothes, even though my height exceeded hers by five inches. I felt like I was

47

stuffed into undersized sweaters and blouses. Dorrie had all the good qualities that I didn't have. She was thoughtful, gentle, calm, unselfish and giving. I was not. She actually liked to be nice with people and benevolently offered to clean the dishes and fold the laundry. I called her a goody-goody, but our sibling rivalry developed into sincere respect when we were in high school.

To me, my family was the most financially challenged of the other neighborhood kids. The big treat we had was membership for tennis at the Concord Country Club, but whereas our peers could order sandwiches and candy, we were restricted to one fifteen-cent cold drink a day. Mine was grape, David's was orange Fanta. We heard cutting remarks about not going to the Arnold's house for lunch because there was only yucky homemade root beer and peanut butter jelly sandwiches.

The Gills had tuna fish, the Moultons had pastries from Sally Ann's food shop and the Springs had absolutely everything. I always felt that the budgetary restrictions tightened the family unit and contributed to our walks around Walden Pond, picnics at Punkatasset and bike rides all over Concord. Yet, wistfully, I would watch the neighborhood kids caravan to summer houses on Cape Cod, while we mowed lawns or washed cars. The highlight of each summer, however, was a precious two weeks in North Haven, Maine.

At the end of August, we packed up the car with food supplies that were carefully spaced around three little sleeping bags for Dorrie, Wendy and David. The black lab slept on top of all of us. It was 3:30 in the morning and totally dark as we wended our way on empty highways to reach the ferry in Rockland, Maine. We were all so excited! There was something magical about being all together at the early hour. We could hardly wait to see the annual vacation friends with whom we sailed, played tennis and had boating excursions into Mill River. Words can hardly describe how much we loved North Haven, 'fairy path', patches of raspberries, the log cabin and the boat house that always smelled like sweet pine and varnish.

I cherish the memories of high school at Concord Academy, which had an all-girl population of half boarders and half day students, like me. I never felt the absence of guys, however, because of our fraternal affection for all the

49

neighborhood friends. I was kind of an average student, majoring in getting into trouble and varsity sports. The number of times I was told to go to the head mistress, to Mrs. Hall's big green chair, exceed how many fingers and toes I had. Academics were not important to me when I could spend time skateboarding, playing lacrosse or singing in the Concord Academy Choir.

My very best friend at CA was Mia. We both were seventeen and shared a lust for life. We were inseparable. Mia was from Middleburg, Virginia, and we spent wonderful vacations and Thanksgivings at her home. Middleburg was big on riding, so we'd get on horses and gallop through the fields on 'steeple chases'. To be honest, I was always scared to death on these rides, and when Mia wasn't looking, which was always because I was riding behind her, I held for dear life, nearly ripping out the mane of the unfortunate equine.

In our senior year, Mia asked me to come for Thanksgiving dinner at the house of a red-headed friend, Monty. Monty was a couple of years younger than we were and was so wealthy he had the entire second floor of his family's mansion to himself.

Mia and I arrived to the formal family gathering on horseback, our faces and clothes all spattered with mud. Mia still sat down for the meal, and of course I followed. We had a premeditated game in mind—we would only eat food that was white. So, our plates were covered with white cauliflower, white creamed onions and white potatoes. We giggled through the entire meal. That's the way we were, a pair of jokers.

I played ridiculous games at Concord, too, and now wonder why they meant so much to me then. For example, our geometry teacher was a Miss Graffam. I'd arrive at seven o'clock in the morning, pull down the great big graph for geometry and write with an indelible two-inch-wide magic marker, 'Graph 'em with Graffam,' which I thought was hilarious. When Miss Graffam saw the vandalism, she looked directly at me and demanded that, once again, I take a walk to the green chair and Mrs. Hall, the Head Mistress.

Another prank was inflicted on our algebra teacher, Mrs. Coogan. She had a classroom that was level with the ground, and one hot day in spring, when there were about twenty of us in class, we decided to 'test' Mrs. C.

51

Whenever she would go to the blackboard to write something, I'd coordinate and orchestrate which of my classmates would jump out a window. Every time Mrs. C. was at the board, I'd point to a couple of kids, and out they'd go.

Then Mrs. C. would turn back to the class but not notice anything, although two or three girls were gone. When she'd go to write on the board again, I'd get two more to jump. Turning back one time, she said, "There's something different in this classroom," but went to write again, so I had more kids jumping, until finally just Hilly Baldwin and I were left. Finally, Mrs. C. turned and, looking very confused, reiterated, "I *know* there's something different in this class. Where are the other students?" Hilly and I sat there with very straight faces, saying nothing.

When it came time to graduate, in '65, the college advisor really discouraged me, saying, "You certainly don't have the academic acumen to get into any good four year college or university. I think you should major in physical education." She put me down because I really wasn't interested in school work, so I applied to five junior colleges and, probably to the advisor's chagrin, got into all of them. I chose Centenary College in New Jersey because it was close to where Mia would be attending the Philadelphia College of Art.

Although my focus had been on practical jokes and varsity sports, Concord is one of the best prep schools on the east coast, with an exemplary faculty. My advisor, Jim Parker, a history teacher, was a wonderful man. He was always a very kind, understanding and supportive mentor, despite my mediocre grades. We had an ongoing joke. Whenever I later received recognition from a Minister of Health or an important government official in my international travels for HIV/AIDS prevention, I would send Jim a postcard and jokingly write, "Not bad for the B-minus kid, huh?" Regretfully, Jim had a stroke and died in 2013.

College, Marriage, Divorce

At Centenary College I got stuck in one of their far-off dorms, Spence Hall, a little house off-campus. Mum and Dad had taken me to the college, bringing along our little black Lab, 'Revie.' I remember vividly—after I got everything up to my third-floor room—watching them drive away down the street in the old Ford station wagon, Mum and Dad and the black Lab, and I just started weeping. I was terribly homesick already.

I hardly ever had to study at Centenary. I'd get into dirty-dog double dares about taking a chemistry test without opening a book, and I'd still ace the test, probably because Concord had prepared me so well. I was majoring in chemistry and when I got into classes of qualitative chemistry we had to take unknown solutions and figure out what they were with algorithmic chemical analyses. So, if you burned something and it was green, then it was barium, do this and that and it was something else.

One time I was given some stuff in a lab, smelled it and thought, 'This is nail polish remover, like the Revlon product I had in my room'. Five minutes into the class I explained to Dr. Hedges, "This unknown solution is acetone. I've taken it through all the tests," which was a dirty filthy lie. Dr. Hedges asked, "How could you possibly have researched the product so quickly – you just got it?" But sure enough it was acetone, identified because of the familiar smell, and I left the lab headed for the tennis court. I graduated with high honors, because of common sense, and was president of the student council. Centenary was a breeze for me.

I had a Concord neighborhood friend, Bucky, and he and I were like brother and sister. One day he invited me to drive down to North Carolina for a weekend to see his very good friend Kim, who was going to the university there. Kim had a date, and I was Bucky's 'date.' That evening, however, Bucky had too much to drink and pretty much faded out. Now I felt abandoned and was totally bored. With time, I started talking with Kim, and he seemed like a really nice guy.

The next weekend Kim drove all the way to New

Jersey to see me at Centenary. After that, he often came up from Chapel Hill, and we'd always have a great time. Since he was from Manchester, less than forty miles from Concord, we were together a lot during the summer too. He'd come visit me from Camp Monadnock and was adored by the family. He was a wonderful fellow, with a great sense of humor, and he seemed to really care about me.

When I finished my two years at Centenary, I went on to the University of Colorado, in Boulder, selected because it was in the mountains and I liked skiing. Since I was a chemistry major, I was able to plan my labs for Tuesday afternoons and Thursday mornings, which meant that Thursday afternoon through Monday night I went skiing. I'd take off every weekend for Vail and mountains beyond. Kim would come to visit periodically, and I was really falling for the guy.

In the spring of 1968, I took a leave of absence from the university, moved to Boston, and on December 7, Kim and I were married at my parents' house in Concord. It seemed like the right thing to do. Back in 1968 you sort of had this fear that if you didn't marry by age twenty-one you'd never get married—you could end up like my seventh grade teacher, an aged spinster who lived on Old Mill Hill. And, to be honest, there was a part of me where I could hardly wait to set up my own house and live independently. So I probably got married more with the idea of being married than with being in love with Kim.

We lived in Boston, and I worked at Harvard Medical School's Department of Surgical Research doing liver and kidney transplants on abandoned dogs. Although the dogs were treated with great care, there is no way I could do research on these wonderful canines now because they are now so very dear to me. In Boston, I happily played 'Harriet-Housewife' with Kim while trying to get pregnant, but there were infertility complications. These challenges continued when we moved back to Boulder for me to finish my BS.

I clearly remember returning one time to the OBGYN doctor's office in Boulder after he had done a series of fertility tests the day before. He looked me directly in the eye and said, "You'll have trouble having babies, if *you ever do.*" To me, that was like someone shoving a tennis ball down my throat. I was horrified with the news. It meant I had let down not only my family but the family of Kim as well. I began taking fertility pills and getting injections of human gonadotropin (HCG), all of which made me feel awful and none of which worked.

Just before I was to graduate from Boulder, my academic advisor told me, "You are lacking 4 credits; you need to take microbiology to get your BS degree." This was in April, and I was supposed to graduate in May. I didn't want to spend the summer taking just one class so I talked to the professor of microbiology, and I asked, "Could I take the final exam, and if I do well enough, pass-fail, could I get the credits?"

He was not happy and rationalized, "You haven't taken the labs, you don't even know the difference between a bacteria and a fungus. You don't know parasitology, you don't know virology, in fact, you don't know anything!" But I begged, "Let me try the exam," and he finally gave in. I bought one of the Cliff Notes books on microbiology, read every word, pretty much memorized the definitions, took copious notes, and, to the professor's chagrin, passed the exam. So I did get the credits, I did graduate, in the spring of '71, with a 4.0.

Kim and I then moved to Washington D.C. Still trying to get pregnant, I went to a doctor on K Street. They did an ovarian biopsy and found that 'there were eggs present', but they weren't mature. There was still hope?

In a post-surgical checkup, I remember walking out of his office into the parking lot feeling desperately alone, in tears, and as I was going to my little yellow station wagon, a big limousine drove into the parking lot. I didn't even see who was in it because I was crying so hard. Then Sammy Davis, Jr. jumped out and as he approached me asked, "Why are you so sad?" There I was, an emotionally crushed twenty-three-year-old, and I returned his stare, while blurting out, "I can't have children and having babies is really important to me and I'm just failing everyone and what good is life?"

He stayed with me for about fifteen minutes and remarked, "Look, there are lots of other things you can do. You're still young, you've still got your whole life ahead of you, there's so much you can do." I listened to Sammy and marveled at how such a small-statured person could have all this wisdom. I finally broke the solemn mood with, "I've *got* to get your autograph. No one will believe I had this conversation with you." I found a little piece of paper and he wrote 'Sammy Davis, Jr.' on it. This definitely cheered me up a bit because I had been grasping for straws, and here was an important man trying to help me.

The infertility phase of my life was a very difficult time for me. I remember moments in supermarkets where every baby I saw brought me to tears. I was obsessed with having children. I compared the obsession to having a big duck with floppy webbed feet hanging from my neck. I could be happy about something, and in one second my mood could change when I remembered the infertility dilemma.

At this time I was working at the Institute for Behavioral Genetics in Boulder, and my research was going well. It could be a good day, and then, ugh, there's something on my neck, oh yes, that darned duck with big webbed feet. The fact was that I'm infertile, I'm sterile, I'm all those really bad words.

Looking at this in retrospect, maybe this was all meant to be, for I now have children all over the world. If I had

had my 2.2 kids when I was married to Kim, I wouldn't have been able to devote so much time to the work in HIV/AIDS and certainly would not have been able to do all the international traveling, but I sure didn't see that perspective when I was in my 20s. The infertility situation was one of the reasons my marriage broke up, because I wasn't fulfilling Kim's needs or his family's hope of having grandchildren. Our communication simply fell apart, and five years after we got married, we divorced.

About twenty-five years later there was a fundraiser here in Los Angeles, and I had heard that Sammy Davis, Jr. was going to be honored for his incredible contribution to theatre. I was very curious to try to see him and thank him for his words of encouragement back in 1971.

With no expectations, I drove to the Century Plaza Hotel with the cherished piece of paper with his autograph that I had very carefully saved. And then I saw him, surrounded by his entourage of people. Quite timidly, I approached the group and excused myself for interfering with their evening conversation.

Standing right next to him, I mustered the courage to

say, "Sammy Davis, Jr., so many years ago you gave me such hope when I was really depressed after a doctor's appointment. You really improved my morale with your healthy perspective of what is important in life and told me that even though I couldn't have kids that I could still have a happy future."

There, I said it, and now I felt like a jerk realizing there is no way he could have remembered me. But he studied me with his infamous rectangular Sammy Davis, Jr. smile, and he said, "You're the little girl who was in Washington." I melted.

Stanford, Harvard, UCLA

While I was working at the Institute for Behavioral Genetics in Boulder, Colorado, I was told about a woman in the Department of Pharmacology at Stanford Medical School who was studying alcohol and barbiturate dependence in mice. I was told she was the source for medical ridicule because her way of testing the mice's withdrawal from alcohol was to pick up a mouse by its tail, spin it slightly, then mark different degrees of the convulsions to determine exactly what level of dependence the mouse was displaying.

When I moved out to California, I decided to check out this researcher, just for the heck of it. I wasn't working, was in the middle of separating from Kim, and was getting pretty bored after wandering around San Francisco for two weeks. At that point I was staying with a former roommate and just to get out of her hair I drove down to Stanford to meet this doctor. Well, it turned out Dr. Goldstein was not a kook and she was looking for someone to help her with the research, so I spent the next two-and-a-half years of my life getting mice drunk and dependent on alcohol.

Now, it's not all that easy to get a mouse drunk. You can't just give a mouse alcohol because they don't like the taste, won't drink and won't get drunk. I needed to be creative! So I designed little mouse cages, removed all of their food and replaced it with the diet drink chocolate Slender – they didn't like strawberry – laced with alcohol. Basically, I was starving the little critters and making them ravenous for my alcoholic concoction! The mouse would drink the solution, because it was the only food available, then would proceed to get a little wobbly, and ultimately be so fall-down drunk that he couldn't even drink the Slender.

So, that didn't work, nor did infusing alcohol into the abdominal cavity of the mouse, but we finally succeeded with an alcohol vapor box, in which the mouse had no choice but to breathe in the ethanol. We had to maintain a specific level of blood alcohol for three days to get the mouse dependent. Then we could take him through withdrawal and determine what was biochemically happening to his little brain. I thought it was cool stuff.

One of the highlights of my tenure at Stanford was the significant amount of tennis that I played with the Stanford Women's team. Then, after tennis, I would stretch at Angell's Field, the running track beside the tennis courts. It's not that I enjoyed stretching so much as it was that I could socialize with a group of runners called the 'Angell Field Ancients'. I was 26 and these fellows weren't exactly ancient – perhaps in their 40s.

As I was filled with energy and effervescence, I was asked by some football players if I could be the mascot for the next game. The guy who was usually the 'tree' was out of town. I jumped at the chance and was the mascot for the football team for four games. It was an absolute hoot! The tree is still the mascot of Stanford.

However, I missed my family and so moved back to Boston. I found a job at Harvard Medical School, this time in the study of anti-fertility agents in ground squirrels. I worked with a renowned researcher, Dr. Don Fawcett, giving the ground squirrels fertility drugs and then seeing what was actually happening histologically with their reproductive cells and spermatozoa. After two years, I was getting bored with laboratory medical research and concluded, "Enough, I've had it with mice, I've had it with rats, I'm sick of doing nasty things to little furry animals."

I decided to go into Public Health. I'd always had an interest in medicine and health promotion and I loved trying to help somebody who's down, either emotionally or psychologically. I wanted to find out how people's attitudes and behaviors relate to medicine, disease prevention and health promotion.

Since I worked right next to the Harvard School of Public Health, I had the chance to talk to several students. Now, in order to be accepted into any graduate school, one has to take the Graduate Record Examination (GRE). That created a bit of a problem for me.

Back in my Stanford days, I had no intention of ever going to graduate school. I was pretty happy just plodding along in biochemical medical research, playing tennis and being the mascot-tree for the football team. But I once again got tangled up in a dirty-dog double-dare.

I had a friend, Tom Nelson, who was very interested in

seeing what would happen to the GRE score if somebody took the test and just arbitrarily entered the answers – *a-b-a-b-a-c-b-b-b-c-a-a*, whatever. So I did just that and my reward was a dinner at a favorite restaurant. I filled in the little blanks randomly for the Math and English and whatever other sections there were. When the results came back, my score was 350. A pathetic score but I didn't care. 350 for someone who hadn't even read the questions? Now it was on my record that my GRE score was 350 out of 800.

But…when I wanted to get into Harvard School of Public Health, they wanted the GRE scores. It was public information that I had already taken it, resulting in the pathetic 350. I went to the admissions office, and they said, "Unacceptable—there's no way you can be admitted with that score. You can't even be accepted as a special student with a score like that."

Now, in my mind of logic, answering the GRE questions is ridiculous. 'The white house is to the black house as a penguin is to a rat.' 'All of the above.' 'None of the above.' 'It's only A if B is nonexistent." And who cares, anyway? I was never any good at standardized tests.

But now it was time to get serious, so I took the Kaplan GRE course and studied really hard.

This time around my total was 720, which out of 800 was okay. I got my score, went back to Harvard admissions and talked to the Director of Admissions, a really nice man, Chuck Campbell. Chuck looked at my 350, then my 720, and said, "Who took the second test?" I said I took it. He said, "There's no way someone can dramatically increase the score like that."

So I told a little white lie. I explained, "Well, the first test I took"—there was no way I was going to admit that I got onto a dirty-dog double-dare and just went in there and immaturely filled in all the blanks without reading the questions—"I was going through a very terrible divorce and my mind just wasn't on it, and psychologically and emotionally I just was vacant."

Chuck bought my story, and I was accepted by the Harvard School of Public Health in 1979. Most of the students were on a 'pass-fail' system. They made it quite clear to me that all they really wanted was to get a degree from Harvard, they just wanted the name and status. But like a nerd, I was actually there to learn about the medical consequences of behaviors and attitudes. After most of the classes, everyone was gone, there were no further discussions or study groups. Bummer. Perhaps it was time to move on.

I snooped around, looking at other graduate schools in Public Health. My friend Vivian recommended that I check out UCLA. I discovered that UCLA had a fine program in Behavioral Sciences and Health Education, so I applied to the School of Public Health, was accepted, and moved to Los Angeles in 1980. I was there for two years and was enthralled. After classes we had study groups, we had special projects, we did community outreach work. I loved the school—and still love it.

But I always felt that my transfer from Harvard to Los Angeles caused a schism in my relationship with Dad. Dad was a Harvard man, and anything west of the Charles River was like a no-man's land. And then there was the reputation of Los Angeles, where we New Englanders believed L.A. was a Mecca for flakos, druggies, hippies, rejects and losers. But I swallowed the jabs and actually found that most of my Los Angeles friends were also transplants from the East Coast. I know Dad was equally disappointed when his grandson and my Godson attended Berkeley instead of his Cambridge alma mater.

After graduation, I worked at the UCLA Jonsson Cancer Center, under the mentorship of a woman who is still my role model, Helene Brown. I went in there on independent research, studied adolescent risk-taking behaviors and did a literature study on what contributed to child abuse, teenage pregnancy, and alcoholism in teenagers. Through this reading it became clear to me that the concept of peer education was an effective strategy for modifying risk-taking behaviors.

It was now '81-'82. I was finishing my studies at Jonsson, completing my report, and that's when I met Steve. Meeting him gave me the awareness of what the AIDS situation was. How could anyone treat a person like Dr. Steve the way they were—why were people treating him like a leper? And why was there such an issue about homosexuality, when it's a non-issue?

L.A. to Paris

It's said that you have to be in the right place at the right time for opportunity to come knocking. In my case, I was in the wrong place at a bad time when opportunity kicked in my front door.

In 1985 I began to work at AIDS Project Los Angeles (APLA). After extensive interviews and discussions I was hired by an absolutely wonderful man, John Mortimer. John wanted me to work in the Education Department in a new position as Community Outreach Coordinator. One of my ideas was to establish a Speaker's Bureau with people who were infected and affected by HIV/AIDS, "What a great way to educate the public—personal testimonies and experiences of those who live with the disease!"

As the Community Outreach Coordinator, I set up the Speaker's Bureau with professional and paraprofessional volunteers from HIV/AIDS-related organizations. It was an incredible group of physicians, nurses, counselors, teachers, pastors, actors, celebrities, and so many wonderful people who were personally influenced by the AIDS epidemic. For most of the members, the Speakers' Bureau was like a psychological support group. We shared personal stories that ranged from spirituality, medical information, communication skills, presentation strategies, as well as sadness, apprehension, and fears. In 1985, AIDS was a death sentence. There were only a few who lived more than a couple of years.

Our group met every second Wednesday of the month, from four to six p.m. Our outreach activities took us into schools, religious organizations, corporations, businesses, law firms and probation homes for youth. We were proud of our accomplishments in providing information on the medical definitions of HIV/AIDS, transmission, prevention, and poignant stories of living with HIV/AIDS. I also took great pleasure in baking brownies or cookies for our 'family' of thirty to thirty-five, and after our discussions we often went to a local restaurant or café for dinner and coffee. We were a very close group, united by our feelings of anguish, discrimination and hope.

Then a new administrator was hired as Director of

Education for APLA. He was quite the macho male, and I could tell immediately that he didn't like me. He just didn't. Right off the bat, he told me I couldn't have another Speaker's Bureau meeting until *he* could attend. I implored, "I'll videotape the meeting for you. This is really great support for the members: I have them practice presentations, and it's just very, very important for them."

But Daniel said, "No, *listen* to me—you can't do it. *I* won't be there." There were uncomfortable disputes for two months, and I was walking on egg-shells. I suddenly had a sense of, "Maybe this job isn't working out."

Then one Friday night I was staying late at the office and got a call from someone who needed five hundred Spanish AIDS brochures at Belmont High right away. How could I possibly get them five hundred Spanish brochures so quickly, particularly on Friday when everyone else was gone? So I called a friend who worked for L.A. County and said, "Hey, O.C., bail me out. I'll take you to lunch next week if you can help me with this," to which he replied, "No problem." And everything worked out just fine.

When I got back to the office on Monday, however, I learned that someone had called and said, "We want to thank Wendy Arnold for all she did, getting us five hundred Spanish brochures on such short notice—you got yourself a really fine person there."

That's all Mr. Administrator needed. He came to me and said, "You *didn't* requisition the brochures, you *didn't* do *this*, you didn't do A–Z," and I thought, "This is getting worse and worse."

I felt I was close to getting fired, since he kept saying the word, "Insubordination," because he thought I was just acting up. For example, I was putting in extra hours, but he wanted me out by five. Sometimes that's not possible. So, all of that had me thinking, "This is not good. Maybe I don't want to be in a large organization with someone telling me what to do."

While this was going on at APLA, an article about me and my work was published in a March 1987 *View* section of *The Los Angeles Times*. A photograph with the article showed me at a small school in West Hollywood, surrounded by six or eight youth who seemed entranced with the information I was sharing with them. Needless to say, there had been very little discussion about sexuality in this school, let alone any mention of AIDS.

Late one evening I got a call from a woman who said her name was Madame Line Renaud. With her thick French accent Line explained that she was the director of an organization called *L'Association des Artistes Contre le SIDA (L'AACS)* in Paris. Little did I know that in the French AIDS community Line Renaud was the Liz Taylor of France! Line was presently in Los Angeles, said she'd read the *L.A. Times* article about me, my outreach activities, and how I was mobilizing youth to be peer educators. She wanted to meet and discuss the possibility of having me set up a similar program in Paris.

Before Line returned home, we spent many hours working on a grant proposal for Madame Michelle Barzach, the Minister of Health at that time. We discussed goals and objectives, how we would recruit the Parisian youth, how we would conduct the trainings, and where we could take our youth peer educators. Line Renaud was very enthusiastic about the novel concept of peer education and was optimistic about getting both government and private financial support.

Meanwhile, I was put on probationary warning at APLA for my 'insubordination' and for being too close and friendly with the Speakers' Bureau volunteers. Too close? They actually *were* my best friends, since so many of my acquaintances away from work had discouraged me from their social circles because of my immersion in AIDS, the gay community, grief and death. But Mr. Administrator told me I should have an entirely professional relationship with the speakers and volunteers. By then I was pretty upset with the conflicts between us and his interference in my personal life.

It finally was recommended that, "You take your good work elsewhere." So I was fired for reasons that to this day still make no sense to me! A mid-May Friday was my last work day. A great many APLA volunteers, clients, all the speakers and terrific staff members were giving me a farewell party on that afternoon when the receptionist tapped my shoulder and said there was an urgent phone call for me. I told her, in front of everyone, to give it to the guy who'd gotten me canned, but then said, "Never mind, I'll get it," and I picked up the phone.

"Bonjour, Wendy Arnold, c'est Madame Line Renaud de Paris." She jubilantly told me that the proposal we had worked on had been accepted. She wanted me in Paris by August. So, I was unemployed for maybe four and a half minutes.

I went up to that administrator, who by now I disliked intensely, and I gave him a big kiss on the lips and said, "Thank you for being such an asshole. Now I can do what I really want to do."

Then I began my preparations for France. I already could speak a little French, "Je parles un peu de francais," "la plume de ma tante"—I could even sing some French songs! I spoke 'franglais,' describing the weather and how lovely the day was. But it was clear that this would not be sufficient for my employment as director of an educational program sponsored by the French Ministry of Health. I decided I needed an intensive course in French and applied for tutoring at the Berlitz School in Los Angeles.

As part of the intake process, I was interviewed by an

adorable man named Jacques, who needed to assess my current level of French conversation and my reasons for learning French. So I told him I had to learn some pretty esoteric words, phrases and medical definitions because I was going to be doing AIDS prevention in France, and there wouldn't be much of, "This is a beautiful day."

So Jacques asked, "What kind of esoteric French?"

"How do you say in French, 'If there are cuts and lesions on the penis, this could be dangerous for HIV and AIDS?'"

"Oh, mon Dieu," he blurted out and immediately *pulled* me into his office, obviously afraid that others in the school had heard what I'd said.

For the next several weeks, I memorized phrases describing "les moyens de la transmission du VIH", "la prevention," "quelques activites sexuels." By the time I packed up for the six months of work in Paris, I was pretty good in conversational French – as it related to HIV and AIDS! But that was all, other topics were missed.

Once in Paris, I sounded quite knowledgeable in French

when describing the urgency of educating Parisian youth about taking precautions to avoid exposure to HIV and why adolescents are at particularly high risk for HIV/AIDS. I knew all the idioms and technical terms and felt pretty confident with the subject matter until…one evening

I was invited with Line Renaud to have dinner with President Jacques Chirac and his wife, Bernadette. For the first fifteen minutes of conversation I was doing *just fine*, talking about my work, reeling off HIV/AIDS statistics in France, describing the development of the "Training Manual" and presenting our prospective goals for a peer education program for the youth of France.

But when I finished talking about the HIV and AIDS topics, President Chirac asked more questions, this time about my family in Boston, my education, the politics of the United States—and I couldn't say *a thing*. I just sat there looking pathetic. I didn't know the ordinary French words for any of that. I only knew how to talk about AIDS. Nor was that the only time I got into hot water with my French.

Once things were really moving well, I was invited to Nantes in Southern France to talk about the program's progress and success. I was again with Line Renaud, who always drew the media—with coverage from Radio France and French television—and lots of politicians and celebrities. At the evening press conference, there was a huge audience of more than two thousand people. With cameras flashing and videos recording, I was invited to the podium to share "L'experience Americaine: the new program in HIV/AIDS prevention for youth."

Filled with importance and 'bien assuree' because I had lived in Paris now for three months and really knew my stuff, I was talking about the importance of choices for youth and strategies of empowerment—that we need to give all the information, all of the alternatives, to let young people decide how to make their own healthy sexual choices.

So, churning out the memorized phrases learned from Jacques at Berlitz, I was describing that we don't ever want to isolate young people who have decided *not* to have sex, those who are still abstinent and are still virgins. We don't want these kids to feel any differently than those who have had sex as this was one of the objectives of the Peer Education Program in Paris, which by now was called *L'Association Jeunes Information SIDA (L'AJIS)*.

I was telling the audience that, in fact, when I was married at twenty-one years of age, I was a young virgin— what I said in French was, *"Quand j'etait mariee, j'etait une petite verge."*

And everybody started laughing. I didn't see what was so funny—I thought, with my Boston morality, that being a virgin was a really good thing. As I spoke, and they giggled, I thought about Nan Nan, my maternal grandmother, who was one of my absolute role models. I knew that she would have been proud of me for confessing my virginity before marriage in front of all these people and yet the audience was just *roaring* with laughter.

I looked over at Renan Velly, a colleague, and asked him, in French, "Why are they all laughing at me? Did I say something wrong?"

And he said, "Wendy, il y a grand différence entre *verge* et *vierge*."

What I'd said in front of these two thousand people was *not* that "when I married I was a young *virgin*," but that "when I married I was a young *penis*." Because *vierge* is the word for virgin and *verge* is the word for penis.

France also was where I had my first exposure to a different culture. There were moments that were particularly uncomfortable for me, like how to hold a staff meeting. I was familiar with very punctual, orderly and concise meetings. It wasn't like this in Paris.

I arrived in August, but it wasn't until mid-October that we had our first staff meeting with Line Renaud and several other people I had never seen before. The meeting was scheduled for four o'clock, but people just started wandering in at six. Then they all wanted a glass of wine, nobody was introduced, and there was no agenda. It certainly was different from any meeting *I'd* ever attended, and I was *really* frustrated that nothing was accomplished.

When I returned to my hotel I called my dad and said, "Dad, you're not going to believe the staff meeting I just went to," then described what had taken place. He laughed and replied, "The French have been like that for centuries,

so don't think you're going to change them in six months."
And that taught me a very important lesson about having
realistic expectations about what I can do when immersed
in a different country. Now I realized, "Ah, you know
what? I'm not going to sweat this disorganization because
I *can't* change the culture. Now I have to learn to adapt *my*
work, my agenda and my ambitions to *their* culture."

Although I love France, it was very difficult for me to
live there, since there was quite a bit of anti-Americanism
in '87–'88, particularly as it related to AIDS. Sometimes I
would find a dead pigeon just outside my tiny office—the
dead pigeon symbolizing *l'Americane que commencé
fleau*, since at that time the French thought AIDS had
originated in the United States and that we were
responsible for its spread throughout the world.

However, that experience in France was the start of my
work in international HIV/AIDS prevention, and I will
always be indebted to the kindness and trust of Madame
Line Renaud for inviting me to Paris.

PEP/LA

Youth peer educators are a powerful, energetic, resourceful, enthusiastic, motivated, unprejudiced, unbiased and clean-slated population. The concept of using peer education in HIV/AIDS was obvious to me. I was able to grab it and run with it, knowing it would be a successful strategy for discussing sensitive issues like sexuality. Looking back, it was like Gestalt therapist Fritz Perls' comment, "Don't push the river—it flows by itself."

After I set up the Speaker's Bureau in 1985 at *APLA*, I was at the Hertz Middle School in West Hollywood talking to the teenagers about risk-taking behaviors and explaining that many teens get into drugs and alcohol, which really mess up judgment.

Then I asked the group, "What do *you* think are some of the reasons why teenagers are at getting infected with HIV, the virus of AIDS?"

Their response: "Well, *we* have sex because it feels good. *We* have sex because everybody else is doing it. *We* have sex because it seems to be the thing to do. *We* have sex because we're curious and horny."

So instead of *me* saying, "You have sex because___," *they* were giving me all the right responses and were using the word 'we'. That's when the light came on, a Eureka moment, as I told them, "You know what, *you* should be the ones doing this education! How would you like to help me reach other students your age, so that we can do HIV/AIDS prevention through peer education?"

A couple replied, "Yeah, that would be fun, that would be really neat, and we need community service hours." So I gathered some students from Hertz High School, got parental consent and gave them just very basic information along with some suggestions for communication. With our handmade posters, we carpooled to nearby schools to introduce teenagers to the dangers of HIV/AIDS.

It was immediately obvious that they were the most effective means for not only recruiting additional teens but also for reaching them. "Hey, guys, you know, I'm a peer educator in AIDS prevention and I'm doing it for community service. We really want you to join our program because it's really fun to meet other kids like this. And I know that I'm making a difference because last week somebody said, 'Wow, I didn't know that!' So, I have a lot of cool information, and you can do this too." The ball was rolling and the ripple effect multiplied the number of kids involved!

As the only teens, the first peer educators loved coming to the Speaker's Bureau meetings and meeting the other members. Some were initially cautious about meeting a person with HIV/AIDS but they quickly learned that these fears were not justified. They fit right in, interacting with doctors, nurses, lawyers and people from very diverse backgrounds. They particularly enjoyed the actors from soap operas and movies. When they returned to their respective schools with stories of the meetings and outreach activities, more and more teens joined us.

After I left the Speaker's Bureau and *APLA*, went to France and came back, I worked for about one year with another nonprofit organization called the *Adolescent*

Alliance, which was run by a very sweet woman who just didn't know anything about management.

The concept of the *Adolescent Alliance* was setting up a group home for homeless and runaway troubled teens with HIV/AIDS. The Executive Director was a therapist in marriage and family therapy and she wanted to run the psychological component for the six kids who would be coming into the group home. I was to be responsible for the HIV/AIDS information both at the house and in the community. So we had two basic components: the in-home care and educational outreach.

The Director's idea of raising money was hoping she could win the lottery, although she never bought a ticket. In 1989, we got a grant from the *Centers for Disease Control*. Now we could furnish the group home, get our license and develop educational resources once *the funds were received*. The money was promised in September so Fef, the Director, happily went out to buy beds, refrigerators, computers, and more. She even, prematurely, hired two assistants to help with all the plans and materials, but September came and went as did October, November and December. As it turned out, Fef, didn't have a clue about budgeting or finances, so within a short period of time we were bankrupt.

This was my last straw. It was also the impetus for me to break away and independently set up my own non-profit organization. I had no inkling of how to do this, but I gathered up some of the teen volunteers, found a tiny space for an office and called the new agency the *Peer Education Program of Los Angeles (PEPLA)*. We received our non-profit, 501(c)(3) tax-exempt status in 1991.

However, there was a real Catch 22. When you're just starting up an organization and you apply for a grant to any foundation or funding source, nobody wants to fund you, because you're brand new. They want to see a track record. To prospective donors, I would write the mission, goals, and evaluation, and they responded, "There's no way one person will be able to do all the training, outreach, data tabulation and program maintenance," to which I responded, "I'm already doing it." The fact was that I had set up realistic and reachable objectives that really were not hard to meet. But people really didn't want to put money into PEP/LA without a history of maintaining income and revenue.

Anyhow, that's pretty much how I started with youth, and I think it's because I just love their energy and enthusiasm. Also my high school years were my favorites—I had a ball in high school, so I guess mentally I kind of identify with them. I'm just a big teen. I used to go to their basketball games and family dinners. I write letters of recommendation for the kids in the program to go to college and then continue to provide recommendations once they get out of college, for jobs. That's actually a large component of my activity with them, continuing to help them out.

On Wednesday afternoons I'd do street outreach, sometimes in Venice. A guy named 'Jonesy' ran a junkyard, and I'd meet homeless and runaway kids there, talking to them informally about the dangers of drugs and AIDS. They called me the 'Condom Lady' because I had a large rubber condom hat and I had made a condom necklace around my shoulders. I'd go down there with some of the HIV-positive people in my speaker's bureau who had been formerly incarcerated and were recovering drug addicts. They were street smart and had a message of tough love – 'don't follow the path of destruction that I took: stay out of gangs and stay away from drugs'. It was the concept of peer education that reached the youth with vital life-saving messages.

One time, maybe in '92, I was at the junkyard with my friend Jonathan, and as we were leaving, somebody jumped out and knifed me in my thigh saying, "Gringo, we don't like white people around here. Get out of our neighborhood and mind your own business." I grimaced, "I'm doing AIDS prevention with homeless teenagers over in Jonesy's junkyard," but he answered, "We don't like you here." He stuck his knife right in my butt and I told him, "Take that out," and he finally jerked the knife out. Then Jonathan—I don't know where Jonathan went, I think he took off— just left me right there, and it was like hello, he was supposed to be like a bodyguard?

Then the guy asked, "What's in your bag?"

I guess he thought I was undercover, out to find the drug dealers and their customers. I knew it was a notoriously bad area because there were little 'gatekeepers', kids who whistled to warn the residents when an outsider was approaching the neighborhood. But I still wanted to try to get to the runaway youth in the junkyard and let them know there were programs to help them off the streets and give them help with their dependence on drugs. This was right on Third Avenue in Venice.

So the guy with the knife repeated, "What's in your bag?" I opened the bag in front of him and poured the contents out on to the street. "This is bleach for cleaning needles and syringes, these are condoms and I'm doing AIDS prevention. Here's my card. I'm just trying to get people involved in an AIDS prevention program."

Before I went to Daniel Freeman Hospital for medical help, I mentioned that I needed some getting into this neighborhood. I was hoping some of the locals would join my educational outreach in HIV/AIDS prevention. Much to my surprise, the rather scrappy looking fellow replied, "Yes, I'd like to help you."

Here's this guy who just knifed me—it was a small knife, one of those Swiss Army Knives—but I said, "Well, I think I'll go to the doctor first, but why don't we meet at some place on Lincoln Boulevard, like a coffee shop? I'll meet you next Wednesday at four o'clock." Sure enough, he was there and for several weeks he escorted me through the streets of Venice. We were not overly successful in getting the residents to talk with us, but I left several packets of bleach, water and lots of condoms for him to share with others at a more appropriate time.

As the memories of working on the streets of Venice flood my mind I cannot help but think about another drug outreach activity, this time it was in the shooting galleries of Puerto Rico, around 1991. They call these locations 'shooting galleries' because it's a gathering of drug addicts and dealers who are actively injecting or 'shooting' heroin and crack.

I was invited by the Harvard Institute for International Development to establish a peer education program for case workers at the San Juan AIDS Institute. I was to train case managers to reach drug addicts in a grim ghetto called 'La Perla'. Now, I really wasn't the appropriate person to be the principal investigator of this project because I have never even used drugs and was repulsed with the idea of 'shooting' drugs into my veins. However, once again, I *chose* to take the challenge and boarded the plane for Puerto Rico.

The thirty-five case workers were receptive to the discussions in HIV/AIDS education through peer education. They were all recovering addicts and certainly knew the psychological, emotional, physiological and physical demands of drug use. I was honest about my substance abuse naiveté yet looked forward to sharing a bunch of innovative strategies for individual and group counseling.

Our descent into La Perla was announced by the 'gate keepers' who whistled warnings like little birds. I was with Katherine who was a missionary from a Catholic agency. The slope steepened and darkened into subterranean alleys. We finally reached an open space that was like a small outdoor theatre with wobbly wooden benches. There was only a murmur of conversation between the hunched figures.

Katherine introduced me to a woman who was originally from Detroit and had come to Puerto Rico for the Mecca of drugs. Denise looked like an old 'bag lady', but I was told she was only 23. She looked up at me with a sullen and empty stare while she tugged at a sheet of scab on her right calf. The opened wound bled extensively with the tearing but there was a bucket to catch the flow of blood. Then with intense deliberation, Denise unloaded the syringe with heroin, stabbing the needle directly into the gaping and gushing hole.

I could not find words to speak. To put it mildly, I was horrified with this action and numbly stared at the earthen floor for what seemed like an eternity. I was awakened to reality when the missionary nudged me with, "Tell Denise about your program in peer education."

But I digress – let me get back to L.A. In addition to the work in Venice, I also did street outreach on Hollywood Boulevard. The kids ignored me at first, but when I befriended some 'leaders', luring them with hotdogs and cokes, others would join our group discussions. I'd also put them into food lines for the homeless at La Brea and Santa Monica at five o'clock.

Still, with these kids, it was "fuckin' this and fuckin' that, and you don't fuckin' have to fuck" – it was every other word out of their mouths! I'd never heard it used as a noun, adjective, adverb and article all in one sentence! And believe me, when you're around that kind of language, you start using it too—I mean, "What the fuck do you mean by that?" It just flows freely.

One time, after my mouth was just whirling around with their language, I went back to my office on Wilshire. Just as I got in and put down my little condom bag, the phone rang. Without thinking, the first words out of my mouth were, "How may I fuckin' help you?"

"This is Sharon Sinclair from the LA Unified School District. I'm looking for Wendy Arnold." And I suddenly realized what I'd said. So, with some ridiculous accent, I quickly replied, "Well, I'm one of the street outreach workers. I'll give her a message that you called." I put down the phone and thought, "Well, I really screwed up that one."

There was a similar incident when the phone rang one day and somebody said, "This is Alice from the Mickey Mouse Club in Florida." I thought it was a friend pulling a prank, because it was like eight o'clock at night—who's going to be calling me that late saying they're from the Mickey Mouse Club?

So I sang, "M-I-C-K-E-Y-M-O-U-S-E," and she said, "No, I really am from the Mickey Mouse Club and we'd like to have some of your peer educators come down here and talk with the 'peanut gallery'. We're going to have a special day in AIDS prevention for teens."

Laughing totally out loud with this joke, I still thought a friend was pulling my leg, so I continued, "Meeska, Mooska, Mouseketeer, Mouse Cartoon Time now is here!"

She questioned, "Is this Wendy Arnold?"

I came back with, "Is this Donald Duck?" I just went on. How much more of a jerk could I be?

"Well, this really is Alice Robbins from the Mickey Mouse Club and Buffalo Bill Bob and the Peanut Gallery and all of that," she told me, "and actually I got your name from the CDC. They kind of warned me you were a little on the goofy side, and you're certainly living up to my expectations."

I finally asked, "Are you really calling from the Mickey

Mouse Club?" It turned out that she wanted, and would pay for, one of the PEP/LA peer educators and a parent to go down to Florida, be part of a youth forum. So one of the teens, Joshua, and his parents went down and just had an absolutely wonderful time.

Penguins

I have more than 10,000 penguins in my house. There
are penguin tooth brush holder, cups, mugs, wastebaskets
and of course those made of crystal, glass, metal and fluff.
Stuffed penguins hide behind plants, sofas and gardens.
They range in size from 3 mm to 6 feet. I've been
collecting these flightless birds since I was around ten. It is
very easy to find a present for Wendy, as I always
appreciate yet again another penguin. The game is to find
one that I don't already have. I've been known to stop
traffic in Ghana upon seeing an inflatable penguin on the
side of the road. There are penguin treasures throughout
Thailand, the Philippines and even China.

There's one very special homemade penguin I got
when I was in Omsk, Siberia. The Mayor of Omsk found
out that I liked penguins and requisitioned one of her staff
members to make one for me. Apparently the woman went
into her closet and started whacking away at a bunch of

Russian furs and leather items. The final product looked more like an owl than a penguin but the note from the Mayor is very precious to me.

The penguin is the mascot of PEP/LA because the penguin has many characteristics that I think are exemplary of a good peer education program and of a youth peer educator. First of all, penguins are very *adaptable*. There are seventeen different species of penguins. Some are the little rockhoppers in the Falklands, some are in South America, some of the little blue penguins (fairy penguins) are in New Zealand, then you've got chinstrap, and there are penguins all over the world. They adapt to their environment, particularly those guys up in Antarctica who try to incubate their little frozen eggs.

We all have to be resilient and flexible, we have to adapt our message to whatever population is at hand, with respect to their demographics, age and backgrounds. Again, this is the concept of peer education. I recall one time regretting that I had agreed to speak at a gay organization of Asian men. I was not appropriate, as I was not gay nor was I Asian nor was I male. I didn't identify with their very personal issues. I try to match the PEP/LA speakers to the specific concerns and issues of our target groups.

A second characteristic of penguins is that they're *monogamous*. When mama penguin and papa penguin mate, they stay together for all seventeen years of their life – a novel idea. After the egg is laid and transferred to the male, the female escapes to the ocean to finally feed. Now the male loses 40% of his body weight as he patiently waits for his mate to return. Then, quite cleverly, they hook up to raise the chick together. If one of them dies, that's it – mateless for life.

A third characteristic is that penguins negotiate, they know how to *compromise*. Papa penguin builds a nest for mama and throws in fish heads and shells and a couple of rocks. Mama comes, looks at that and says, "You know, the rocks are fine, but that fish head and this shell, they gotta go. It really ruins the décor of this nest." Papa penguin replies, "I'll tell you what, I really like that shell, so here's what we'll do"—and they literally toss it back and forth. Finally mama will say, "Okay, we're gonna put the shell back in but the fish head, that's out," and papa penguin says, "Okay, fine."

As educators, we have to compromise with the local traditions, cultures and values. The Africans are notorious for being late. A training that is to start at 8 a.m. never sees more than half of the participants before noon. The agenda I had planned for the first day is shot, now I'm four hours behind.

Those are just some silly reasons why penguins are the mascot. There are penguins on the PEP/LA brochures, training manuals and website. The real reason is that penguins are just so darn cute, and it's fun to be anthropomorphic about them!

Newroads High School

A sunshiny, scrubbed-sky morning has wrapped itself around Santa Monica. Set back from the north side of broad Olympic Boulevard, deep inside the enclosed Newroads High School compound, well over a hundred students are gathered on the small circular school commons. Some are draped on the benches of half a dozen weathered blue-green metal picnic tables. Other teens have flung themselves randomly to the ground onto long blue sheets of plastic in the center of the lawn. A few students lounge on the relative luxury of folding chairs, the rest stand in nonchalant groupings of studied indifference around the perimeter. Backpacks squat everywhere. A babble of young voices ripples softly through the cool air.

It's 8:05 a.m. of a February Wednesday, and Wendy is due shortly to make four presentations to some of this group. She and PEP/LA won't be alone, though. Six other organizations will also be speaking during the day, not only about AIDS, but also about planned parenthood, sexuality, teen dating violence, drugs and alcohol, eating disorders, and other teen issues. Now a quartet of New Roads peer counselors climbs onto a slightly raised porch at the front of the crowd and begin to announce the order of the day, talking—one at a time—through a standing mike. The teen speakers don't look totally comfortable addressing their peers but pretend they are.

The tableau turns into a swirling flow of bodies as students start heading to their assigned rooms. Wendy still hasn't arrived. The last few students drift out of sight, leaving three adult counselors who walk briskly back and forth across the now empty common.

At 8:32 Wendy appears. She's wearing a light green turtleneck sweater with a white and red AIDS ribbon patch on it, pinstriped charcoal pants, sensible black flats, and a large wool handbag with a shoulder strap. Trailing behind her are two male Afro-American PEP teen counselors, one, Juwan, tall and sturdy enough to be an L.A. Lakers guard, dressed in black sweats, the other, Maurice, skinny, a broken jaw wired together, wearing small silver-framed glasses, cream shirt and tan slacks. They are carrying cardboard posters.

"Good Morning," Wendy announces brightly to her hosts. It's obvious she's set her energy level to its usual "high" position, despite the morning hour. "Where do we go?"

She and her crew are quickly led to a dance rehearsal room, one wall covered with mirrors, two other walls with parallel bars bolted to them. Only seven teens are present, which doesn't faze Wendy at all. She and her two PEP volunteers start taping the colorful instructional posters onto one wall. Finished, the two young men sit down in white plastic chairs facing their audience, and Wendy flings herself into her presentation. The students quickly focus on her, intently watching and listening.

Within moments, she's roped them in with her casual, irreverent approach. The students glance around to see if it's OK to grin or laugh, realize it is, and broad smiles crease their faces when Wendy zings them. Having set them up, she knocks them down, as she starts to speak about alcohol, teen date violence, and AIDS. "Go on,

Juwan," she says to the tall PEP counselor, "tell them about Sara getting raped."

Juwan first speaks about himself having had an STD thirteen months ago, which he got from his girl friend, the mother of his child. He then recounts that a young woman recently had had too much to drink at a party, had passed out, and waking had found she had been raped in a limo, with no idea of who had done it. Now, she'll have to wait for up to six months to find out whether or not her rapist was HIV positive, and whether she also is. Drinking can be dangerous, Juwan ends, coming down hard with, "AIDS is not the way you want to go out." This is one serious young man. He does not joke.

Wendy reaches down to the floor and picks up two cardboard posters, to which are attached dozens of photographs, all of relatively young individuals. "These are my friends," she says, "All were infected, a lot of them are dead. I stopped counting how many friends have died when I reached two hundred, years ago. Let me tell you, I'm getting really sick of this disease. I've been watching people die for twenty-two years. There were around 1,600 known HIV cases in the U.S. when I started in '82. Now

105

there are almost 900,000. Something's got to be done to stop this epidemic."

Three more students drift into the room, listen with serious faces.

Wendy now swings into her routine of basic AIDS information: the three ways to get HIV, four body fluids that carry the virus. "We've got to talk about sex, if we're going to talk about AIDS," she throws in, mentions pre-cum and turns it into a joke. "You know that a basketball player first dribbles before he shoots. Well, so does a guy having sex." The students laugh. She's got them. "OK, pre-cum has the HIV virus too, not just semen, so you're not safe if the guy pulls out before coming. You can get pregnant like that, too," she adds.

"How many of you want kids?" she challenges. Most raise their hands. "Well, don't get infected—your baby can get it from you." She talks back and forth with the students about each topic, both her face and body always animated, moving almost like a fencer across the smooth dance floor, her eyes fixing on one student face after another, trying to bore into their minds.

A girl sitting on the floor, her back slumped against the rear wall of the room, repeatedly responds to Wendy's questions and statements. She wears an off-white cloche hat, dusty orange sweater, knitted white scarf, designer blue jeans, and pink sneakers. Innocent oval face, wide-open blue eyes, and thick blond braids. She looks about seventeen, doesn't seem to be the intellectual type, but she's sharp. She keeps pushing her verbal ping pong with Wendy.

As the forty-five-minute presentation draws to a close, Wendy asks if anyone would like to volunteer for PEP/LA. Sure enough, the girl with the cloche hat raises her hand. Wendy is delighted. The girl agrees to take part in a PEP presentation the following morning, if the school will let her out. Wendy reels in her catch. She and the girl huddle at the back wall as the other students saunter out.

Five minutes later, a second group of teens meanders in, this time twenty-five to thirty strong. The group dynamics are different, but Wendy adjusts to the change, launches into her core presentation again. Suddenly she stops dead, "How many people here know someone living with HIV or AIDS?" she asks. Almost half of the students raise their hands. There is a moment of stunned silence.

Then Wendy lunges forward, races on again, as two more PEP/LA volunteers, white girls dressed in casual clothes, slip in quietly behind her, stand next to the AIDS posters. Noticing, Wendy immediately involves these volunteers. The girls giggle nervously, push their backs against the wall behind them, but rattle off hard facts about HIV infection.

The second presentation flows on, finally ends with applause. Two down, two to go. Wendy is on a roll, as always.

Courts and Offenders

I also have frequent appointments with the court system, talking with people who have been picked up either for lewd behavior, solicitation or prostitution. Around '85, I was on assignment with Judge Larry Rubin of the 3rd District Court in Santa Monica. He had met me at one of my presentations to the Santa Monica City Council. He called requesting me to talk to a young sex worker about the dangers of prostitution and drug addiction as they relate to HIV and AIDS.

During the following two hours I made it clear that I was there to educate her about the medical issues and was not a determinant to her court offense. It was a very personal and embarrassing discussion on how difficult it was to determine if one of her 'johns' could be infected with HIV. She wrongly assumed that AIDS was only in gay men who were frightfully symptomatic and sick. She admitted that the money she made from prostitution was to support her drug use. We also discussed how drugs were clearly associated with risk-taking behaviors.

She decided that she wanted to see if she had been infected with HIV. The HIV antibody test was brand new in 1985 and there was a lot of skepticism to its reliability. With time, it would be mandatory for offenders of sex crimes to be tested. The young woman was unaware that there could be an exposure through oral sex. She listened and showed her appreciation for the session with a hug. The time had been worthwhile.

I met with Judge Larry soon thereafter, and he asked me what we should do with this court offender. Now I was to be part of her sentencing? I recommended an outpatient drug treatment program, as she had two infants at home. I said, "How about, if when people are brought in, as a condition of their probation or sentence, there is mandatory AIDS education, and they have a mandatory HIV antibody test," and he said, "I like that a lot." Since then I've been meeting with court referrals.

My work with court offenders has taken me to March 2014 with my assignments with the Los Angeles Police

Department (LAPD). Detective Bill had a novel idea of setting up a Prostitute Diversion Program where men who have been picked up for soliciting prostitutes, or who are themselves 'pimps', can attend a full day seminar on the legal consequences of having a prostitution charge on your record. They also hear from former prostitutes about the dangers of picking up women. It's similar to the concept of traffic school where if you attend the full day course you will get the conviction removed. We are pretty proud of the fact that more than 700 men have gone through our program and there are only four repeat offenders.

My responsibility in this seminar is the discussion of how prostitution can lead to an exposure to HIV. As I am still in a wheel chair from all the knee infections and seventeen operations at St. John's Hospital, one of my caretakers will prop me on a table in front of the approximately sixty participants. It is quite the motley group of young, old, professionals, blue color workers, transgender, cross dressers and diverse cultures. Lee provides simultaneous translation into Spanish for more than 65% of the attendees.

As there are frequent breaks for the men to walk

111

outside to a mobile van for mandatory HIV testing, I will often start up a conversation yearning for the lugubrious details of how they were apprehended! Most are caught by 'sting prostitutes', who are actually undercover cops. Apparently, as soon as the solicitor-john mentions any monetary amount in exchange for a sexual act, the decoy alerts the nearby patrol cars, setting off piercing sirens and flashing lights. It all sounds very dramatic and I have asked if I could be a decoy but, first, I'm afraid no one would stop for a sixty-six-year-old woman in a wheel chair and, second, Detective Bill says it's much too dangerous to be in these situations.

One time during my discussion on HIV transmission, I locked eyes with Burt, a friend of mine from my sports club. Naughty Burt, naughty indeed! I reassured him that of course his secret will remain confidential.

Let me go back to 1990 and Judge Rubin's court system when a woman, Cynthia, was apprehended and behind bars in a jail cell. I was to talk with her from the adjacent corridor which would mean raising my voice for her to hear. I explained, "Judge Rubin, I don't feel it is appropriate or even effective for me to discuss personal behavior when we have a barrier of bars between us. Let me go sit with her."

But that concerned him, "No, no, she's an offender, she's a felon, she could be dangerous. We don't know that much about her."

So I said, "Look, you've got guards here."

He finally asked, "You're willing to go in there?"

I said I was, so in I went and sat closely beside her. It was a very endearing eye-to-eye conversation where we analyzed very sensitive issues. As I am an advocate of decriminalizing prostitution, I listened empathetically and nonjudgmentally to her reasons for being a sex worker.

This is the oldest profession available to women, particularly the disenfranchised, and it is sex between consenting adults. When it is illegal, women are isolated from their children while they are imprisoned and can be quite vicious when released. Now, granted there is a different story for each offender, but this young woman convincing described how she needed money to buy food for her baby. Or, like a gullible idiot, I believed Cynthia's rationale for soliciting 'johns', the men who seek prostitutes.

One of my ways of reaching people like her, as with the work I've done abroad during interventions to prostitutes, freelance sex workers and commercial sex workers, is the strategy of displacing the consequences of a faulty action and transferring them to another, like a family member or close friend.

I asked Cynthia to tell me more about her baby and if she had a boy friend. With her eyes focused on a paper in her lap, she whispered that her three month old baby was her life and there was nothing more cherished than having the suckling infant at her breast. I continued, "Well, how would you feel if you transmitted the AIDS virus to the baby through breast feeding?" She was silent. "I didn't know that could happen," she blurted out. She basically knew very little about HIV/AIDS rationalizing, like so many others, that she wasn't a gay man and 'didn't shoot up'. It was the same dilemma of denial where women simply did not feel at risk.

I stayed with Cynthia for two hours, encouraging her to

get tested and providing specific information on proper condom use. She made it very clear that she was going to continue as a prostitute. It was an easy and lucrative business. I made her very aware of the legal consequences of getting caught a second time when it would be a mandatory prison sentence. I knew my limitations as an educator and couldn't get her to change her profession.

I've also used the displacement strategy with men who drive trucks in India and Africa as they see many prostitutes on the roadways, then bring the virus back to their wives. "Do you love your children?" "Yes, very much," they respond. I elaborate, "If you got infected, progressed to AIDS and got very sick, who'd be the 'Baba' of your children?" And then they respond, "I hadn't really thought about it like that."

For years, I've had some very interesting experiences meeting with these 'court people'. They came to my office where I consciously left my door open a little bit because I had no idea who they were and often I met with them after hours. It was dangerous only one time—once again, making a choice.

Sometimes these discussions got pretty entertaining! For example, there was Melanie, another prostitute, who was in a revolving door between the courts and the streets. She made it very clear that she was not going to stop soliciting men. The money was too good, she could make $2,000 in one evening. What she did with her body was not my concern, it was her business. My goal was to talk with these 'colorful' people from the public health perspective to avoid an exposure to HIV. Hence, there was more emphasis on risk-reduction with condom use.

I decided I would teach Melanie how to put a condom on a man with her mouth because many of her johns are drunk when she is propositioned. I figured she could just slip it on with her tongue. The only prop I had in my office to teach her was a candle, so I was demonstrating how to put a condom on the candle with her mouth.

That's when the postman walked in…. So here was Melanie with the candle in her mouth, and I'm saying, "No, no, you start by holding the shaft, and then…." I'm being very graphic—but the postman's eyes…!

Sometimes I ask offenders for ten dollars, or whatever

they can donate, for the class. This would make it more professional. I questioned one woman, "When was the last time you had unprotected sex?" She told me, "Girl, two hours ago—I needed the money to pay for this class."

Then there was another time I made an appointment with a man and requested when we talked by telephone that he bring his court case violation number. They were still coming to me for the mandatory AIDS education.

The man, I'll call him Mr. Rogers, told me he'd picked up a prostitute who was actually a cop, and, of course, as soon as the decoy asks, "How much money are you willing to pay," or, "How much money do you have in your pocket," the mention of a dollar amount justified an arrest. Then the flashing lights from a hidden police car, the 'whoop' of the siren and the locking of handcuffs as the 'john' is busted. So Mr. Rogers had been picked up for soliciting a female cop.

When he came into my office, I couldn't believe my eyes. I looked at him and said, "Mr. Rogers, could I see your driver's license?" Because I wanted to make sure his name matched the case violation number, and it did.

He was eighty-five years old!

I said, "Mr. Rogers, you're *eighty-five years old* and you're *still* out there? Don't you realize how dangerous this could be?" He just smiled. Working with the court system is still very rewarding.

L.A. Court Referrals

One early morning I was conducting a "Train the Trainers" with self-described 'blue collar' employees in the Department of Water and Power. They were relentlessly accusatory with, "Oh AIDS is just in the gay community and for drug addicts who share their 'works'. We're not gay, we don't shoot up drugs, so get off our case, we don't need to do this!"

They continued, "Well, you, Wendy, are obviously gay or you wouldn't be this committed to the AIDS epidemic." And I replied, "That's not the issue. This is not a gay disease. This is a sexual disease." But they kept jumping on me, "You're denying it, girl, you're denying it. You're gay and all your best friends are gay." I finally told them, "I know this will come as a real disappointment for you guys, but I'm not gay. I'm committed to this because I do have a lot of friends, gay and non-gay, who are dying from AIDS."

119

They just want to blame somebody, and that gets me angry. Whether it's by ethnicity or sexual orientation or background, they want to avoid any responsibility to change their personal behavior. I don't think we can do that. Finally, I have to say—and repeat it like a broken record—"I'm sorry you feel that way, I'm sorry you feel that way, I'm sorry you feel that way."

What I try to point out is that AIDS is a disease, not a disgrace. AIDS is a medical and not a sociological concern. When the subject of AIDS is introduced, one immediately thinks of sex, 'dirty sex' and promiscuous sex. Somehow we've got to get over that barrier, because we can't talk about AIDS without talking about sex, and nobody wants to talk about sex. That goes right back to the reasons why we should start this education at a younger age.

I got my first 'information' from my parents, and my Dad mixed me up so much when I tried to talk to him about sex. I don't remember how old I was, maybe seven, and I asked, "Dad, I've heard about sex. What is sex, and what does it feel like?" Dad immediately said, "Go ask your mother." But Mum wasn't there, lucky for Mum. Dad said, "Well, sex is very comfortable, it's like shaking hands." And that was a good enough answer for me.

Almost on cue, the doorbell rang, and I went to see who it was. It was our neighbor, Mr. Gill, and Mr. Gill said, "Hi, Wendy," and put his hand out to shake my hand, and I said, "Oh, Mr. Gill, I don't want to have sex with you." And babies arrived if you put a large net outside the window and waited for a stork to drop in an infant. That's the kind of sex education I had. There was no sex education.

Then when people don't talk about it, it gets more irresponsible, more dangerous, and you think of sex as either this big novelty, this curiosity, or it's dirty and it's dangerous, and that contributes to experimentation because you know that you shouldn't try it. I also feel that 'sex education' is a misnomer and *sexuality* education' is more accurate. Sexuality education brings in the culture, the gender, the mores, the traditions, the values, the family structure, the environment, the demographics.

At some point you also have to have realistic expectations about who you're going to reach. I feel that it is pointless to put scarce resources into a community that wants abstinence only, period, end of paragraph. Providence Catholic High School wanted me to help them set up a peer education program in AIDS prevention, with abstinence as the only solution—I could only talk about abstinence and postponement. I told them I'm not the appropriate person and recommended that they find someone else.

They made it very clear that we could not mention the word 'condom' during the presentation to the whole school. But I always tell the students, "Hey, if any of you want to come up after the discussion to ask us any personal questions, that would be just fine." I make sure, especially with the Catholic schools, to leave an extra fifteen minutes for personal questions, because just as you're about to walk out, "Wendy, I really gotta ask you, when my boyfriend and I were using a condom and it broke—" I mean, the repressed students are often the most experimental. It's the 'Tom Sawyer effect'. Tell them, "Do not have sex," and the first thing they want to do is have sex.

I've mentioned that I worked with the LA Municipal

Court System and the Santa Monica Court System. Offenders, as a condition of their sentence, have to have mandatory AIDS education and frequently they do community service with me. Well, there was one woman, Sondra, who was picked up for doing a little more than just a massage. An undercover cop paged her, made an evening appointment, and went to her massage parlor in Venice. She had no idea who this guy was because she usually has the same clientele.

She was a nationally ranked paddle tennis player, so during her time with PEP/LA we played lots of tennis. After her tennis game, on the day she was arrested, Sondra told me that she rushed home, quickly showered and met the guy at the massage parlor. As she massaged him, getting him to the point where he was clearly aroused, she said, "Do you want me to release you?"

As soon as she said that, the cop jumped up and shouted, "You're under arrest," because from that point on, it's illegal. The description she gave of this cop—aroused, leaping off the massage table with his little soldier between twelve o'clock and three o'clock, running around getting the handcuffs, cuffing her and saying, "You're under arrest." The whole image of the scene she portrayed was just hilarious. Actually, I feel that what two consenting adults do is their business and that prostitution should be legalized. Prostitution is one of the oldest and most lucrative professions. We're not going to change what two consenting adults want to do.

Anyway, Sondra said she could help me out with transportation to the PEP/LA outreach events. She had a big van and could drive some of the peer educators to Flintridge Catholic School, a good two hours away. I warned all the peer educators, the volunteers and the friends with AIDS who were going to help us with this presentation to keep the discussion conservative, keep it down and please watch your language.

When we arrived, there was a team of nuns and sisters to greet us. In spite of the words of caution, the very first exclamation from Sondra as she dismounted from the van, were, "Jesus, fucking Christ, I can't believe how far away this place is!" I told her, "Sondra, keep it down, keep it down." She finally simmered down. That was one immediate demerit against us, because she'd used the Lord's name in vain, so we all went in quite intimidated.

We did our basic information and, yes, I talked about abstinence until I was blue in the face. But there is a trick when in Catholic schools where we can't mention the word 'condom.' But we are told that if one of the students in the audience mentions 'condom', that is out of our control and can be justified. So we talk about the importance of abstinence, it's not only what the Pope decries but postponing sex really is the best choice. I mean, yes, it is the best way to avoid HIV, but it's 'Pollyanna'; it's like merely waving a wand over sexually curious teenagers and hoping they agree. It's really not practical.

Our ploy is to then ask the students, "Hey, if any of you know of any older brothers or sisters or if you have friends who have made the choice to have sex—everyone has a choice—if you know of anyone sexually active, what would you recommend to avoid an exposure to HIV?" A little hand went up way in the back. His answer was a whisper.

"Excuse me? Could you say that again, please?"

"A condom."

"That is exactly right—and what kind?"

125

"A latex condom."

So the kids are now aware of one viable alternative, as *they* are the ones providing the information. I haven't said anything, I have not used the word 'condom'. You can see all the administrators turning kind of purple, because here we are talking about HIV prevention using a barrier—but PEP/LA has not mentioned the word 'condom.'

There are ways of getting around using what the church says are controversial words. I can make it quite clear when I'm talking to religious leaders—as a Christian, yes, I was brought up in a loose understanding but a respect for Christianity—I let the Christian leaders know, yes, I believe in the Ten Commandments, and one of those Ten is 'Thou Shalt Not Kill'. And if a husband has AIDS and wants to have sex with his wife, they have to use a condom, because if he doesn't, he could be killing her.

I talk about a condom not as a barrier to life, not as a barrier to procreation but as a barrier to death and disease. And the response is often, "You know, that sounds all right." But I do feel that the Church is more open about this now. When I'm invited into a church setting, it is important to do an impromptu needs assessment, asking, "Is it all right to talk about this, may I talk about that? What are my guidelines, what are their concerns, what is acceptable and what should I avoid?" If you don't follow the guidelines, you just don't get invited back, and there's no point in angering people.

I think that as educators we need to know our limitations, know that we're just not going to reach all the people all the time. If you can reach three out of a group of thirty probation gang substance-abusing youth, congratulations! We simply need to show people they have choices and teach people to make their own decisions. Let *them* weigh the advantages and the disadvantages, the costs, the benefits of their actions. Then choose.

Friends

Nancy

My friend Nancy had been living with AIDS for about eleven years. She didn't find out until she was four-and-a-half months pregnant and knowing there was a chance of infecting her baby all she could do in 1990 was to pray that everything was going to be okay.

She was told she could have a late abortion but was afraid to tell her husband because he was, in her words, some 'big old meat cleaver guy'. She was scared to death of telling him, so she didn't say anything about it to anybody. She decided not to have the abortion, she kept the baby, and the baby was born antibody positive.

In the early 1990s, it was well documented that an infected mother passed the virus to her baby at a 30% transmission rate, either during pregnancy, during birth or through breast feeding. Now we know most babies are infected at birth because they are exposed to maternal fluids. As a result, if a mother has a C-section, the transmission can be reduced to 10% and even to 1-2% with the administration of the anti-retrovirals (ARVs) during gestation and at birth. In the USA, an HIV-positive pregnant woman is given the ARVs as soon as they detect HIV.

It was interesting to see that at the maternity clinic I visited in Mutengene, Cameroon, all babies were delivered by C-section, they just assumed the mother was HIV-positive. Nancy was not aware a baby is born with the mother's immune system. So, the baby can be born with the mother's HIV antibodies but not the virus, because the antibodies are in the immune system for the first 18-24 months of life.

In Suriname, South America there were horror stories about mothers who discarded their HIV-positive babies into the bush for the animals. They didn't want to deal with a baby that would soon die from AIDS.

I am reminded of another incident that took place in Suriname. This experience lends importance to what I call 'the Anatomy Game', where training participants write down all the slang words they know for the female anatomy, then for the male anatomy and then for sexual acts. Often the words for the anatomy are like reading a menu: cassavas, banana, pudding, and more. The exercise is a good ice-breaker to help the participants get familiar with the jargon used on the streets.

I mean, a teen doesn't say, "Oh yes, I have sexual intercourse with a man's penis" – it's more like, "He put his hoe in my garden," another way of describing having sex. And when a student asks, "Is it risky for him to put the pencil in the pencil sharpener?" and an educator does not understand the question, then we have a responsibility to humble ourselves by simply admitting that we do not understand the language! We are dealing with potentially life-threatening behaviors when we discuss HIV transmission.

Here is why I digressed to communication strategies in discussing sex: Jennifer was a seventeen-year-old peer educator with PEP/Suriname, in Parimaribo City. Verbally, she was very shy; sexually, she was very promiscuous. When Jennifer realized she was pregnant, she decided to have the baby secretly, in the bush. But there were complications when she suffered serious uterine hemorrhaging and vaginal tearing. She wisely decided to consult with a doctor and then would return to the baby.

But when she stood face-to-face with the man, an authority figure, she was too embarrassed to tell him graphically what her medical problem was. She tried to explain that, "She had a problem down there," gesturing with her finger to her vagina. The doctor followed her hand that was pointing to her feet, responding, "You are fine down there", noting that her feet looked fine. "No, no, doctor, I am not fine down there. I am in trouble," she implored. But the doctor stood his conviction and now was impatient. Jennifer tried again to explain her dilemma, this time to the attending assistant, yet now realized the futility of the conversation. She returned to the bush and died with her newborn. Might it be a good idea to have teen peer educators as translators in obgyn clinics? I think so.

During one of the trainings in Uganda, there was a community health care worker who related a belief that the witch doctor could cure a baby of HIV. The mother was to take the HIV-positive baby to the witch doctor for medicinal herbs. These plants were very toxic and would often give the baby severe diarrhea, respiratory problems and skin rashes. But the HIV-positive woman was told to be patient and to return to the clinic to get tested again in six months. This she did, still the baby was HIV-positive.

Now more herbs and more sickness. Some of the babies died during this regimen, and yet if they lived, miraculously, they tested HIV-negative at 18-24 months. Wrongly, the witch doctor was credited for saving the baby when in fact it was that when the infant developed its own immune system the child never had the virus but had only the antibodies, which were now kicked out.

Let's return to Nancy: When her baby tested antibody positive, Nancy thought, "That's it, I'm just going to have to run away. I'm HIV positive, my baby's HIV positive, I'm going to have a baby with AIDS, the baby's going to die, I'm going to die," and she still didn't tell anybody. Then after about a year, she did talk to other women, some of whom said, "Wait, hold on, you know that the baby can be born with the antibodies and not the virus, wait. Wait until eighteen months, wait until twenty-four months."

She tested the baby at nine months, still antibody positive. Then she tested at twenty-two months, and the baby was negative, tested again at twenty-six months, and the baby was still negative. It just gave her such inspiration, such a hope, such a feeling of "Thank you, God," and the child is now eleven years old, cantankerous as all get-out because he is the son of her husband, who was a big old burly guy.

Her husband died. I don't think she ever told him she was HIV positive, she was too intimidated. And he never told her about his HIV status. Whether he knew he had AIDS or not, it was not confirmed. But he got sick with vicious headaches and blackouts. Apparently when he was hospitalized and very close to death, they found out he had a big brain tumor that was AIDS-related. Viral encephalopathy causes intense confusion and delirium.

I frequently hear of situations like Nancy's, where the husband or partner doesn't know his or her HIV status or will not disclose. There's so much fear in telling a partner because the one who is to blame is often not known, and what difference does it really make? "You were the one messing around, you are the one that's going out, I'm not the one that's bringing it into the family."

The blame game. There is a heavy smudge on the truth.

Sharon

Sharon was a lovely friend whose daughter from her first marriage, Geneen, was an eloquent peer educator with PEP/LA. Sharon had been married to Bill for five years and then divorced. One afternoon, Sharon and her mother, who was a social worker, were watching Dan Rather on TV. They became involved in an interview where a frail man was talking about what it was like to be a heterosexual living with AIDS. This was in the late '80s when there was horrendous discrimination and secrecy. The man, with a tightly wrapped red and green scarf, admitted that even his family was unaware that he had AIDS.

Sharon's mother looked at the man on television and exclaimed, "Sharon, isn't that your ex-husband, Bill, talking about having the challenges of AIDS?" Sharon leaned toward the TV and carefully looked at the interviewed man and replied, "Oh, no. First of all, he's much too thin and then second of all, I was married to Bill for five years, and of course he would have told me if he was sick. Yes, my husband was a philanderer but he was in very good physical condition and not skinny like that. Furthermore, in spite of his other women, we had good communication about health issues." But her mother was quick to interrupt her with, "Wait a minute. That scarf around his neck—I gave him that scarf for Christmas."

So Sharon got a little concerned about all this and immediately called Bill, and of course he denied it. He said, "Are you kidding? I would have told you if I had AIDS. That wasn't me on the Dan Rather show. It must have been someone else." Two years later, when he was very sick, he called Sharon and said, "I'm sorry, I have to tell you the truth. I *was* the one interviewed. I'm dying from AIDS complications and I'm calling to say goodbye. I suppose you should be tested."

She had been on oral contraceptives to avoid an unwanted pregnancy. She didn't even think of HIV/AIDS, her husband was not a gay male, neither of them had ever shot up drugs and she had had only a couple of sexual partners. I hear this all the time. Most women are conscientious about pregnancy but not HIV, certainly not from her husband!

Sharon got tested, and, yes, she was positive, and she was positive to the point where she was actually diagnosed with a full-blown AIDS diagnosis, which is defined as having two hundred immunological T cells or less. A healthy person has between eight hundred and twelve hundred T-cells. She had only fifty-six. She was unaware that she had a severely compromised immune system. Sharon had experienced inconveniences such as chronic fatigue, diarrhea and flu-like symptoms but she always had excuses and justifications for the minor problems. "Oh, it was the food I ate last night or of course I'm tired, I didn't sleep well".

One afternoon I went to visit Sharon and questioned why she was profusely sweating; her clothes and bed sheets were soaking wet. She explained that it was due to how hot and stuffy it was in her apartment. I washed her hair, changed her clothes and sheets then within the hour everything was soaking wet again. We later described this as night sweats, another possible symptom of an HIV infection.

There's denial—"it's not my problem"—until they know and love someone who is infected. This is the Catch-22: "I can ignore the possibility of an exposure because I am not the kind of person who could get HIV." A lot of people are infected by the one they truly love, when they actually had sex for intimacy, not because of being promiscuous and having multiple partners. So I just wish that people would get away from pointing fingers at populations they assume are high-risk! This is a sexually-transmitted disease. It doesn't matter if somebody is homosexual, bisexual, heterosexual. That's not relevant. Period. Paragraph.

Sharon's daughter, Geneen, was one of our most precious peer educators, an absolute gem of a girl. She'd speak from the perspective of, "I can imagine what it is like having this disease because I'm living with AIDS, as my mother has AIDS." Her message was very powerful, as a teen talking to other teens. And she shared the daily apprehensions and the fears of, "Oh, Mom, is that a lesion or just a mosquito bite?" The anxiety and unknowns are so hard for the 'affected' people. But Geneen's message was very powerful in allaying the fears of casual contact because she announced, "Of course my mom and I share meals and snuggles and do everything together—you can't get it that way!"

Because the HIV virus is very fragile. Very fragile—it dies immediately outside of the body. And that's one of the reasons why mosquitoes are not carriers. As soon as the virus is in the mosquito, the virus will die, because the mosquito doesn't have the human immune system. The mosquito is not like a flying syringe! It is different from malaria which is a protozoa and *can* live in humans. This is the *human* immuno-deficiency virus, HIV. It's not MIV—*mosquito* immuno-deficiency virus. So even if you slap and there's blood, it's not going to get into the body. The virus will probably already be dead.

Geneen continued her rationale with another reason why HIV is not carried by insects, "Think how many of the elderly or little babies who can't slap mosquitoes, or people who live in swamp areas prevalent with mosquitoes would have AIDS. We also know that in the United States most AIDS cases are in men between the ages of 30 and

39, men who live in big cities, so we simply can't give the mosquito credit for biting only urban men between 30 and 39! That rules out mosquitoes.

"The disadvantage of this is that the virus doesn't grow in other animal species either—in mice, in rats—so it limits animal medical research. If we could get the virus to grow in a laboratory animal, then we could see what kinds of possible vaccines or medicines could wipe it out. But we can't get it to replicate in another animal system, so it's the immuno-deficiency virus for humans only."

This made sense for the teens in front of Geneen. She had, once again, conquered a young audience with her compassion and knowledge.

David

David was hospitalized in Pomona for cerebral opportunistic infections that were giving him severe dementia and confusion. There were multiple tumors from the invasive cancers, and he would often stop mid-sentence to squint from the pain. The CMV retinitis in his left eye necessitated daily injections of the drug foscarnet, put directly into the eye ball. I flinched with the 'squoosh, pop' sound from this horrendous procedure.

When he got progressively worse, the doctors warned me that his death was imminent. Was it time to call his family, with his homophobic Mom condemning his homosexuality and blaming David for his AIDS? David and I discussed this during his infrequent moments of clarity and yes, he really, really wanted to say goodbye to her.

With the help of Rev. Dan Smith and Rev. Steve Pieters, I was armed with verbal ammunition to emphasize the greater importance of the mother-son relationship to the relative insignificance of sexual orientation. I also recruited the wisdom of Brenda whose son, Scott, had died of AIDS. Brenda and a team of mothers had formed a non-profit group called "Mothers of AIDS patients" (MAP). They were remarkably courageous, strong, eloquent and understanding when discussing the emotions when losing a son or daughter to the complications of AIDS.

Together, we got Mrs. Lathrop to buy a bus ticket from Tempe, Arizona to Los Angeles. When I met her at the bus terminal she was adorably dressed, like a little girl attending Sunday school – white gloves, tightly buttoned blouse, conservative suit with a matching hat. As we drove to Pomona, I tried to describe the challenges and anguish that David experienced on a regular basis. She hadn't even talked with him for two years because of the shame of a 'tarnished and evil' son! I quickly changed the subject to her memories of him as a little boy and fortunately, by the time we got there, Mrs. Lathrop had silenced the 'bible-babble' and calmed down.

In anticipation of seeing his Mom after so long, David got the nurses to help him make big signs announcing, *"Welcome Mommie! I love you!"* They brought a cot close to him so he could sleep near her. David was ecstatic. She, too, was crying as she made her way to his hospital bed. Tightly clutched in her hand was a scraggly blue baby blanket. She exclaimed, "This is the blankie that kept you warm on earth. I want you to take it so you can also stay warm in Heaven!" With my eyes filled with tears, I said goodbye and told them I'd be back with breakfast in the morning. I still smile with the image of their hugging.

It was a rude awakening with screams of, "I hate

myself, I hate myself and this AIDS," when I answered the telephone at 5:00 a.m. "David! Are you OK? What happened? Where is your Mom?" I was shaking with apprehensions. David whimpered an answer, "I woke up in the middle of the night and I had to pee and I stood up and I thought I was at the toilet and I..." David had urinated on his mother's face.

There is so much humiliation for a person with AIDS.

Calvin

It was my day off in Dar es Salaam. I had finished a series of non-stop "Train the Trainers" for AIDS in the workplace in the community of Tanga, near the coast. The participants were employees at Katani, Limited, a 'hemp plant', where they made the heavy ropes for freighters and cargo ships. Many of the workers in the business had HIV/AIDS and there were no policies or procedures for protecting these men from isolation and discrimination while they worked the factory machinery.

The managers were laying off anyone they even suspected as living with HIV or those who had a family member who was diagnosed. Here in the USA we have well established guidelines, the 1973 Federal Rehabilitation Act, that prohibit an employee from firing a person based on a medical infirmity, unless it *significantly* interfered with his work skills. The key word, of course, is who determines what is meant by *significantly*.

It would take about thirty minutes to walk from the youth hostel to the coast of Dar. I looked forward to walking independently without the regular Tanzanian escorts. At water's edge, I was happily distracted by a group of fellows playing checkers near where the ferries embark for Zanzibar. I hovered over their game of bottle caps on the makeshift piece of a cardboard box. One guy joked with me and said, "Do you want to play the winner?" Now, I'm really not very good at checkers but I loved the opportunity to make friends! To his surprise, I enthusiastically responded, "Sure!", as I desperately tried to recall some strategies of the game. I sat down on the log bench and practiced my rudimentary Swahili with the players. This was fun!

I was in the middle of my third game, having miraculously won the previous two, and something just did not feel right. It's that itchy feeling and weird aura. The next thing I remembered was seeing the blur of a blue shirt as three men pushed me off the bench exclaiming, "We don't like Americans!" It was not difficult to determine that they were angry Muslims, but they were very different from the Islam friends I had made in Tanga. This was December, 2002—too close to 9/11 and too soon after my hip replacement. I feared doing damage to the new hip and favored my left side as I tumbled several feet from the assault of kicks and relentless pummels.

No one was helping me! Where were my checkers' buddies? They had run away. Then I saw the knife in the hand of the guy in the blue shirt. In that split second I thought, "That's it, that's how I'm going to die!" But instead of attacking me, he cut off my backpack as he continued to kick me and then ran. I lost my camera and some incidentals but there was little money and my passport was left at the hostel. But I was pissed off.

This whole incident lasted perhaps five seconds but for me it was all in slow motion. Then, I had a vision of my maternal grandmother, Nan Nan, in her purple dress. I heard her cry out, "Get up, Poo, Poo, get up!" She called me 'Poo', probably from my favorite childhood story, "Winnie the Poo". I could feel the blood on my face from the kicks as I watched the assailants run further into the ghetto, but with Nan Nan's encouragement, I did get up.

I was so enraged that these jerks got my camera with the photos of the Tanga training that I hobbled after them through the mud and sludge of the slum. Then I met an old man who was next to his broken down cement hut. "Hatari, Muzungu, danger, danger!" And I angrily replied, "I don't care if there is danger, I'm going to find the man who took my camera." I was totally irrational, totally stupid. The man begged, "Muzungu, please leave." So I left. I was still furious and my body was aching. The blood from my face was blocking my vision. Who cares? I wanted my camera.

Across the busy street was the New Africa Hotel that looked pretty nice. I could see some white folks and now I was ready to give up my tough facade of being a resident of Dar to get the supposed comforts of tourists. The guards at the front door were very concerned with my injuries and continued to ask if I was OK.

Although I had no money and it was stifling hot, I asked where I could get a cup of coffee. They pointed to the elevator and told me the restaurant was on the third floor. I knew not to look in the mirrors in the elevator because if I saw all the blood I was afraid I would panic. The restaurant was closed, as it was after 3:00 p.m. The maitre d' said I could sit at the bar and there was a nice server who immediately came up to me.

I put my head in my hands and watched a combination of blood and sweat drip-drip-drip onto the counter. I looked up at him and saw that his name tag had 'Calvin' on it. I asked, "Calvin, are you Christian?" Obviously with the name Calvin, like the Calvin in the Protestant movement in Europe, he responded that he was. There was a sense of relief as I was still wounded by the Muslim attack. I said that I was too and I was in Tanzania to protect Tanzanians from AIDS and now they tried to kill me and I was so confused.

Then I quoted one of my favorite biblical phrases that had been a guiding light for me in previously difficult situations, *"Trust in the Lord with all your heart and acknowledge Him in all thy ways and He will direct thy*

146

path..." And I had taken the wrong path today, and God was not there to help me. Then I lost it. I guess I suddenly felt safe with Calvin there. But I was crying. I pointed to the area across the street, but there was no one there. Now I wondered if he would believe me.

Calvin asked where I was staying and offered to walk back to the hostel with me. I was delighted and tightly held onto his arm as we negotiated the crowded sidewalks. Why was I still angry? When somebody bumped me on my initial route, I extended apologies but now I responded with "Fucker!" Calvin repeatedly cautioned me to slow down but I felt everyone was out to get me. I can be such an idiot.

He walked me all the way back to my hostel and no sooner was I there and had full intentions of introducing my new friend, my angel, to the other guests and Calvin was gone. I had not thanked him enough! I was indebted to this young man for his kindness.

The next day, I left for Kenya, still 'gun shy' from the experience in Dar es Salaam. I would never have news about Calvin again...until three years later when I returned to the New Africa Hotel to research his whereabouts. He was now working in Mbeya, a fifteen hour bus ride away. The Maitre d' still had his number which I called and we joyously exchanged contact information. Ironically, I was invited to Mbeya to conduct HIV/AIDS prevention trainings in 2010. Of course, I met with Calvin, and we have remained solid friends ever since.

Deanna

At age fifteen, Deanna was invited to San Francisco to visit her aunt. She couldn't wait to get some time away from the family and the pressures of Palos Verdes High School. While her aunt worked, Deanna explored Fisherman's Wharf and rode around on the trolleys and would then find a little coffee shop for a hot cocoa and some Ghirardelli chocolates. Life was good!

On one of her excursions Deanna 'people watched' when a nice looking man asked if he could sit down with her. Sure, she thought, it would be nice company. They talked for more than two hours and she found he was really very nice as he shared stories about the history of San

Francisco. At one point, she excused herself to use the bathroom but returned for more conversation. Why was she suddenly so sleepy? Her head bobbed with the heaviness of fatigue. Her tongue was thick and now the words were slurred. "I need to go back to my aunt's house," she bleated like a wounded sheep. But this nice man explained that he lived just around the block, and she could go there until she felt better.

Deanna remembers nothing of the trip to his apartment and the rest of the day was a blur. As she mustered energy to get out of bed, she noticed that she was sore in her privates. What? She cried out, "What happened last night? Why is there so pain in her vagina? What is going on?" He responded with a coy smile saying, "You begged me to have sex and so, to make you happy, that's just what we did." Deanna was horrified. "You took advantage of me. You raped me, didn't you?"

But she was interrupted by his claim, "Oh, I just remembered what I wanted to tell you last night, but you were so very sleepy. I have that AIDS disease, but you don't have to worry because you are young and your immune system will fight it off." She was now hysterical as she ran out, slamming the door behind her. It was now clear that he had drugged her cocoa.

Deanna was scared to death about sharing this nightmare with her mother, but she was also scared to death about AIDS. When she told her Mom, there was a tirade of, "You probably asked for it, you little tramp, and you probably are infected. There is a test for people like you, go see for yourself."

It was only one week after the rape. Deanna was totally unaware of the "Window Period" where it can take between 2.5 weeks and 6 months for the immune system to show HIV antibodies, if there is an infection. She did not know that there is no way that the immune system could respond so quickly, if there is an HIV attack. And yet the test was positive! "Oh my God, I have AIDS!" she cried to her mother. To Deanna, there was no difference between being HIV-positive and having an AIDS diagnosis.

For the next three months Deanna ate from disposable paper plates with disposable plastic utensils. Her Mom washed her laundry separately from the other family members and told Deanna to only use paper towels to clean. She did not have *any* information about HIV transmission as it was only 1985 and very little was known. There were no resources, and the Internet was not established.

At school, she finally told Iris, her very best friend, and begged Iris not to tell a soul. But Iris was beside herself trying to keep this secret and figured she needed to vent Deanna's dilemma with one or two other friends. That was all she would do, so confidentiality would *almost* be maintained? But those two told two more who told two more, and now when Deanna walked down the school corridors, the other students flattened themselves against the lockers. She heard whispers of "AIDS, AIDS, AIDS!" She was mortified. She was very alone. She didn't want to live like this.

When she got home that day, her mother and little brother were away. Good. It was time. Deanna reached into the medicine cabinet and grabbed two new razors. It took a lot of strength to slice the razors through her wrists. Moments later, she heard and Mom and brother come through the front door. It only took moments for the ambulance to pick her up and take her to the hospital.

151

Psychiatrists tried to calm the frantic teenager with recommendations for her to repeat the HIV-antibody test. It was now four months after the rape. The results were now negative. What? Again the test, and again the negative results. Deanna explains that this period in her life was even more difficult – was she positive or was she negative? It was deduced the first test result was a false positive. She never had the virus.

Lori

For more than eight years, Lori has been one of the most influential speakers with PEP/LA. Her story of HIV/AIDS infuriates all ages from all groups because it deals with the trust of a loved one.

She shares the challenges of her young life in a dysfunctional, alcoholic family, resulting in her placement in more than seven foster homes. The emotional abuse continued and was complicated by sexual molestations. With time, Lori was inspired by 'Miss Brown' who encouraged her to study hard, resulting in a scholarship at California State University.

As a conscientious student, Lori always saved time in her academic schedule to attend a yearly reggae gathering in Jamaica. With a smile, Lori describes her adventurous life swimming with crocodiles and jumping off cliffs into the warm Jamaican water. One time, just before one of her dives, a reggae musician came up to her exclaiming that she was 'the most beautiful queen' he had ever seen. Now she had had a boyfriend several years prior but this suitor was an Adonis!

He continued his courtship sending her flowers, songs and poems from his international tours. By now she was smitten with his love and devotion. One time he came for a visit and surprised her with a marriage proposal. She explains how romantic he was getting down on one knee expressing his commitment to cherish her for the rest of her life. He explained that she was his true angel and he would never, never let harm get in her way. Lori beams when she describes this golden love affair!

As her fiancé, Lori's Prince Charming questioned why they had to use condoms every time they were intimate. "Are you cheating on me", he would ask, "I am only with you, and we're going to get married, so why do we need these condoms between us?" It made sense to Lori, and her contraceptives would protect her from pregnancy.

Some time went by, Lori expands her story, and she described little inconveniences like flu-like symptoms and a chronic fatigue. But there were always ways to justify these problems, like being exposed to lots of people on buses and a demanding work schedule that led to a mild sleep deprivation. Then there were night sweats but these were rationalized as a way to sweat out the fevers. Then there were body aches, severe coughs and urogenital complications, but who had time or money to go to the doctor when these concerns would probably just go away. But one morning she woke and saw that she had swollen glands in her neck the size of jawbreakers. Now she was worried and finally went to her doctor's office.

Lori submitted to a series of blood tests, as she feared throat cancer was the cause of all those huge 'tumors' on her throat. But it wasn't throat cancer. The doctor told her to please sit down before he told her, "You have tested positive for the AIDS virus". This could not be! She had only two sexual partners in her life and with the first guy, they had used condoms, and with her fiancé, they started out using condoms but they decided to stop as they were about to get married. Then she panicked, "Oh my God, my boyfriend must not know that he has AIDS because he would have told me if he was sick and he could never do anything to hurt me. He said I was his jewel, his angel for life. Oh my God, I have to talk to him!"

Her fiancé quickly came over to her apartment when he heard the fear in her voice. She hysterically told him what she was told in the doctor's office and expected him to be equally as horrified. But what followed wasn't even on her radar. "I know you have AIDS Lori, I gave it to you, I told you I only wanted to be with you for the rest of your life and now nobody will want you." "Besides," he continued, "I have lots of money to take care of us so what does it matter anyway?"

The classroom usually goes silent as Lori discloses her HIV status. Then there are exclamations of anger and fury as to why and how anyone could do this deliberately to such a lovely lady. Wisely, the speaker asks the audience, "Who is really responsible for my HIV/AIDS? He didn't hold a gun to my head and demand unprotected sex, did he?" It was a teaching moment, she could have negotiated condom use or at least request that he got tested before they stopped using condoms, right?

Then Lori reaches over for her lunch box-sized bag asking the audience if they want to see the consequences of her actions. Slowly, methodically, she brings out one bottle of medicine at a time while she describes the vicious side effects of each one. "I start at five in the morning and give myself an injection in the stomach which causes a 'charley horse' cramping, then I take this pill which leads to a violent vomiting, then I take this medicine that gives me a splitting headache, then I take....: She goes on and on, listing the multiple side effects of each medicine necessary to elevate her immune system and/or fight opportunistic infections.

The AIDS-related medicines cost her more than $9,000 each month, a big bite into the budget of Lori and her HIV-negative husband of ten years. She has an extremely difficult regimen for taking it every two hours, or with food or without food, and if she misses even one dose, the virus can build a resistance and the medicine is no longer effective.

The students stir with agitation after Lori's testimony. Once again, she has exceeded my expectations with her eloquence.

Suzanne

Then there was Suzanne, who was from a 'upper class' family living in La Jolla, California, just outside of San Diego. She was an extraordinarily beautiful woman, who admitted having had a gamut of sexual partners—not unusual for an attractive, well-educated, intelligent woman.

No one ever thought about who could be infected – it just wasn't in the cards at that time. There was very little discussion about AIDS in '85, '86. People didn't think about AIDS. And in the '90s everyone believed it was still just a gay disease—"I'm not gay," or "I don't shoot drugs, so why do I need to worry about it?" It was like, "It's not my disease, it's so far away from me, so I don't need to take any precautions. I'm going out with really nice guys, who went to Harvard and drive BMWs. I mean, why do we need to worry about these guys?" It was somebody else's problem, always. There was this constant denial.

When I met Suzanne, she already had an AIDS diagnosis, her immune system was severely compromised by HIV, and she had two opportunistic diseases. This was probably '93 or '94. As with others before, I got very close to her entire family, because what happens with me is that once I get to know the person with AIDS, I soon get close to the whole family—the pets, the goldfish, the relatives— because they become really meaningful friends. My life in AIDS is not a job, it's much deeper. It's like I'm in denial about the fact the person is sick, it's not an issue in our friendship, "Oh, that's right, she's got AIDS." The reality gets pushed to a rear burner.

It was always fun to be with Suzanne. As with Michael, we enjoyed the UCLA Performing Arts for fantastic international dance performances. Suzanne liked the 'bar scene', I did not. She laughed at how uneasy I was talking to 'dorfers', my name for the guys who were trying to hit on us. Actually, it was that the fellows were hitting on *her*, and I was just the tag-a-long! The laughter was therapy for both of us.

On January 15, 1996 I got a call from her dad, "Come to Sherman Oaks Hospital immediately, Wendy." Suzanne had been in a shopping mall with a friend, had an intense headache, collapsed, was in a coma. When she got to the hospital, still in a coma, they found she had a brain tumor that had gone totally undetected, a brain tumor probably caused by the AIDS and associated diseases.

When I arrived at the hospital Suzanne was lying in a bed, and she looked angelic: dark hair gently curled around her face. Her dad, her sister, and an aunt were in the room. I went up to Suzanne, and I clearly remember saying, "Oh, my angel, you're always so beautiful."

I put my hand gently on her right hand, and I could feel it was so cold, so cold to the touch. I just prayed with her and said, "Suzanne, we love you very much. We're all here. We're all fighting for you." And then her father put his hand on top of mine and Suzanne's, and he could feel the tremendous difference in temperature—my hand warm, hers very cold.

And then there was a *piercing* cry. He said, "No!!!!!!" And he looked right into my eyes and asked, "Wendy, how much longer does she have to live?"

I said I didn't know, but I've been with too many people who've died, and I know that the extremities start getting quite cold as they start to slip away. But I wasn't going to tell him that – I had no right to, since some people last a long time while some die immediately.

But to see her father weeping, and to hear his cry, "My baby, honey, don't die! Please, baby, you've got to live! I want you to live...." That was one of the most intense experiences of my life, because I'm very, very close to my dad, and I could see my dad doing the same, if I were to die. It's really hard, imagining Dad screaming like that— Dad, so strong, such a businessman, so efficient. And it was very heart wrenching to hear Suzanne's father cry out and sob.

Three hours after I finally left the hospital, Suzanne died. She was thirty-six.

And I was so filled with rage, I was so filled with rage. I went back to my office and just slammed my hand down on my desk, just kicked things, angry. Angry at society, angry at God, angry at medicine, angry about the

160

epidemic—that no one was doing anything about prevention, no one was talking about it.

I still have marks in my house where I kicked the counter. Yeah, anger, anger—I'm still angry, no doubt, *no doubt*. I'm just angry that not enough is being done, and sometimes I just feel helpless and hopeless because nobody seems to be listening.

And that's where I get my passion and commitment. Seeing my friends die can be very motivating.

Moorpark College

It's morning again. Fog hugs the normally sparkling Los Angeles urban sprawl. It's just after 8:30 a.m., and endless lines of cars jam the many lanes of the 405 freeway. Two miles north looms the 101 interchange, arguably the worst traffic merge in the world. Wendy is impatient. Even after all these years of freeway driving, she can't deal with a ten mile an hour automotive crawl. It's a bigger bother than the rutted dirt roads of Zimbabwe.

Her friend Shelley is with her in the car, so at least they can chat to pass the time, Shelley talking rapid-fire about some meeting she recently attended in Sacramento. She takes a really dim view of the budget mentality of the new California governor, whose first priority has been to cut billions in car registration fees to make rich Republicans happy but who now wants to cap enrollment and benefits for many programs badly needed by the poor,

162

especially medical treatment for the critically ill.

Traffic finally snakes its way onto 101 North, and the car starts to pick up speed. In the distance ahead lie gently rolling hills, in pastel brown and orange hues, almost unbelievably picture-perfect. "I love all those hills," Wendy rhapsodizes, "Aren't they great?" Shelley's mind is still on the action hero in Sacramento. "The governor thinks it's OK for people without money to wait in line for months for cancer and AIDS treatment. Does he think a disease is going to wait for economic recovery?" Shelly is outraged, especially since the muscled actor had run for office as a servant of the people.

Wendy slides her station wagon down an off-ramp, and a few minutes later the car is on the Moorpark College Campus, climbing up a steep incline to a cluster of buildings on a hilltop. The car parked, posters and bags full of visual aids are pulled from the back, and the two women saunter over to the front doors of an auditorium. Wendy immediately corrals one of the young women who are also waiting and starts to question her about which students will be attending the AIDS presentation and why. In a couple of minutes, the double doors fly open, a mass

163

of students streams out, and Wendy and Shelley dive into the academic cave.

As the three-quarter-round-stage classroom theatre begins to fill up with students, Wendy chats with the woman professor in charge of the event as students tape Wendy's large posters to a table and to some chairs on the stage. It's after ten now and time to start, so the professor introduces Wendy, who coyly starts off by saying, "I never know what to say," then laughs and charges into the opening moments of the two and a half hour presentation with a torrent of words, stories and images.

"...Mozambique and writing cards by candlelight, moths flinging themselves onto the flame of the candle and frying themselves....Poverty breeding prostitution, prostitution spreading AIDS....Nine thousand Africans infected every day, seven thousand dying each day....Africans saying AIDS means, 'American Invention to Discourage Sex'....Women who think that 'giving AIDS' means 'giving it away,' believing they can get rid of their AIDS by giving what they have to others—so have lots of sexual partners, that way you'll free yourself of AIDS.... Ignorance, misinformation, tragedy, indifference...."

Dead silence in the auditorium. The students have never heard or seen a presentation like this one. This isn't a class—it's life dragged on stage by its ear, kicking and screaming, flayed and bleeding.

"But there's no problem here in Moorpark College, is there?" Wendy now challenges the students. "No problem, right? Quote, 'I'm a virgin—I've only had oral and anal sex.'" The students smile—it isn't really funny, but it's true—some people do think like that. "But, you know, anal sex is the most dangerous for AIDS transmission...."

"Fifty seven thousand people a year are infected with HIV in the U.S., more than eight hundred eighty thousand have the virus in this country. The AIDS epidemic is spiraling out of control!"

"AND PEOPLE ARE NOT LISTENING!!"

She shocks them with the story of her friend Michael, who finally became blind from AIDS, and "all the medicines they kept giving him, and giving him, and giving him—Do you know that some people are now dying from the medicines, rather than the opportunistic diseases? And people actually don't die of AIDS—they die from all the other things."

Then a video of Wendy working in Zimbabwe, followed by one about young gay men who deliberately "bareback" (use no condoms) so they can get HIV, a very odd phenomenon. "But don't get the idea AIDS is a gay disease. It comes from a virus, it's medical—eleven percent of people now infected are heterosexual. You'll hear about some of that a little later."

Now it's break time, and a student named Eric comes up to Wendy, tells her he wants to start a PEP group at Moorpark College. Wendy is delighted—she's been trying for years to get a student group going up here. Three young women come over and join the conversation. When the break ends, the four announce to the other students that a Moorpark PEP group will be formed.

Time to get personal. Shelley gets up to speak to the students about being HIV Positive. Her story will also be a bombshell. It's another typical Wendy day on the trail.

Shelley

Shelley will always be one of my very best friends. For over ten years she's been instrumental to the success of PEP/LA with her brave sharing of what it's like to live with HIV/AIDS. She's poignant, genuine and fantastically eloquent with audiences of very diverse backgrounds. Teens from probation centers, private schools, group homes, churches and many other establishments hang on her every word. I'll try to capture the highlights of her talk.

"I got infected with HIV because I didn't use condoms!" Clear and crucial words for adolescents who feel impervious to AIDS.

Shelley was originally from upper New York State. Her family life was difficult, with verbal and emotional abuse from her parents. She got heavily into drugs—and had lots of unprotected sex. She didn't care about this new disease called AIDS because she heard it was only in gay men and so not a concern for an educated young woman. She moved to Florida and continued with her somewhat wild and frivolous life style. Life was good and so much fun.

When Shelley went to California, she thought she'd escaped the consequences of the life of sex and drugs. She got married to a musician and ran a karaoke bar. Her voice is angelic. However, for several years Shelley experienced one medical problem after another. Her energy was depleted. After a shower she was too tired to dry off and simply collapsed onto her bed. Her mother-in-law called her lazy and a hypochondriac, but Shelley was truly exhausted.

She developed a severe esophageal problem with so much 'white stuff' that she could hardly swallow. She showed this to her doctor, who immediately stepped backwards, exclaiming, *"Why don't you tell me why you're really here!"* Nonplused, Shelley said that maybe it was an ulcer, but that she was basically clueless. The doctor told her she had a yeast infection. Shelley certainly knew what a yeast infection was, but how did it get into her mouth? The doctor exclaimed that she had a broken down immune system.

"What caused this, who gets oral yeast infections?" Shelley inquired. The doctor held up a finger and explained that little babies didn't have good immune systems, to which Shelley quickly replied that she wasn't a little baby. Then a second finger went up as the doctor said that really old people didn't have good immune systems either. Shelley noted she was only thirty-six years old. Finally, the third finger rose, *"And people who have HIV/AIDS; they have destroyed immune systems because the virus has consumed vital disease-fighting white cells."* For Shelley this was the most preposterous category of all because, once again, she was female, and AIDS was not a concern for heterosexual women.

She waited for a fourth finger and a fourth category, but the doctor had finished speaking. Shelley wondered, *"Where was the 'Shelley category' to explain why she had no immune system?"* She looked at him, and he looked at her. There was a ghastly silence. Then he asked, *"Have you ever been tested for HIV?"* This seemed a ridiculous question to Shelley, because why would she bother when this was not *her* problem?

She took the test. Not only did it come back positive, but she was immediately diagnosed with AIDS. She had only fifty-four T-cells, when a normal count for a healthy person ranged from eight hundred to twelve hundred T-cells. One definition of an AIDS diagnosis is when there are 200 T-cells or less. A second definition can be when there are two or more of the twenty-eight opportunistic infections. I have several friends who had 700 T-Cells and four opportunistic infections or like Mark who had two T-Cells and no associated diseases. Furthermore, Shelley had at least five AIDS-defining opportunistic diseases, with the 'white stuff' identified as esophageal candidiasis. All of the medical problems she'd been having were related to AIDS.

It was a nightmare for the first few years. She became terribly sick, then lost her job, her apartment and her unsympathetic husband. Shelley joined PEP/LA after a consciousness-raising experience at one of the AIDS Conferences in Durban, South Africa.

The 'AIDS medicines,' Anti-Retrovirals (ARVs), have saved her life but endangered her heart, liver and other vital organs. She has bravely put up with lipodystrophy, which pulls the fat from her arms and legs and rudely places it like a barrel on her abdomen, as well as behind her neck, which is 'affectionately' called the 'buffalo hump.'

And yet her beauty, inside and out, minimize these awkward metamorphic changes. She appreciates each and every day and has shared her perspective with all of us who know and love her. She is a true role model and the world is a better place because of her.

Zimbabwe

"Muzungu, Muzungu."

There is a rustling of bushes nearby. Peals of laughter.

"Muzungu, Muzungu."

I'm in Zimbabwe. It's my first time in Africa to do HIV/AIDS prevention, October, 1999.

A man named Chamboko McDonald, director of a very small health clinic in Karoi, had read an article, published in *The Global Health Council Newsletter*, about how I'd created an HIV/AIDS prevention peer education program in the Philippines. Chamboko had written to me to ask if I could possibly set up something similar for him in Zimbabwe. He wrote that he had money, venues and training participants for this program. All I had to do was to arrive to conduct the trainings, one for youth peer educators and one for "Trainers" from multi-disciplinary backgrounds.

As with the other 15 countries in PEP/International in 1999, I made it very clear that the Peer Education Program (PEP) was to be a joint financial endeavor between PEP/LA in Los Angeles and the hosting Zimbabwean communities. I feel this arrangement encourages program maintenance and sustainability when local organizations commit to financial and in-kind contributions. They don't need to do much but providing lunches of cassava or bananas or sadza, their staple made of corn meal, demonstrates that they are serious about the program. I don't want to arrive like Santa Claus with PEP/Zimbabwe pens and metallic buttons because then I question the motivation of the Africans attending the training. They have to earn those American chocolates!

So my responsibility is to find the funds for the airfare, training materials, posters, "Training Manuals", evaluations, awards for the participants, "Certificates of Completion" and presents for the sponsors. *They* have the responsibility to cover meals, local transportation and accommodations. The vehicles are usually a major expense because of the high cost of petrol and the living conditions with the international projects can be pretty challenging but always thrilling.

Speaking of challenging, I am reminded of a visit to Suriname, South America, in 2006, where I was flown to the Amerindian village of Kwamalalosotoe, three hours by a little Cessna from the main city of Paramaribo. Ruben, the pilot, landed in a cleared out area just outside a gathering of 40-50 clay and reed grass huts. Hundreds of dark skinned, scantily clothed children ran up to us, chaotically screaming words of welcome, as our engines sputtered to a stop. There was great excitement because the plane was their only contact with occasional foreigners, the 'outside world', medical provisions and educational supplies, such as text books, pencils and paper.

We were led through tangled vines and banana trees to the Chief who was waiting with his council of five. Ruben, my guide, introduced me, as their special guest and 'expert' in 'AIDS transmission'. Again, there was no differentiation between the virus and disease. I quickly explained that I was not an 'expert' but in 2006 had had at least 24 years experience in the epidemic. I think this clarification was lost in the translation. He spoke Creole

174

and broken English. *"Whaddyahgo-on, howyahdahygo?"* ("What's going on, how do you do?") For the next three hours, we listened to the council members feverishly interrupt each other as they shouted facts describing the devastation of the disease.

I was told that 85% of the 967 villagers over the age of 13 were living with HIV, as estimated by a cross section sample of the population. The 'rapid HIV antibody test' had been performed by the Pan American Health Organization (PAHO) two years earlier. Apparently it took only a couple of visits by several rambunctious male adolescents with prostitutes in Paramaribo City to set off the chain of infections.

The Council members described that young girls in this bush community were raped in silence as they walked the six feet between huts. It was the culture and expected, so there was nothing said. Crude tribal markings were done on infants with one sharp knife using one 'blood bowl'. Twelve year olds were pregnant with their second child. There was no mention of the father and, I was told, many of the children were incestuously conceived.

175

In the Amerindian culture, semen is the seed of men and it is very precious. One drop of wasted semen is like 1,000 drops of wasted blood; the man will get a terrible disease and his penis will fall off. There was no way to promote condom use with the deposition of semen into a latex sock!

To make matters worse, there was no refuse or garbage in Kwamalalosotoe, so the idea of promoting condom use and proper disposal of a used condoms was not practical. I was stymied thinking of solutions to decrease the rising number of HIV infections. All I could come up with was 'risk reduction'—was it possible to reduce the number of sexual partners? Could we encourage the girls to shout their disapproval of the rapes? Can we bring in trash receptacles for condoms and other discards? We cannot change culture but how can we modify risk-taking behaviors? In my mind, none of these alternatives carried any significance.

With the darkness of evening fast upon us, the women gathered wood for a community bonfire. We were to leave soon, with the frustration of having provided no solutions. Accompanied by the patter of a muffled drum, the Chief offered Ruben and me a vial of a vinegar-smelling fluid that he poured from a wooden chalice-shaped vessel. Ruben wisely did not drink because he was the pilot on duty. The fermented fruit juice burned my lips as I took one tiny sip. That was all, thank you, now I have to pretend I take more.

Then a woman with a loosely draped cloth and pendulous breasts handed me a ceramic saucer of something that, in the shadows, looked like a mixture of some kind of root and twigs. Again, only a small bite as I determined, but it was not confirmed, that the food resembled crunchy black beetles. I could only yearn for pizza and a burger!

Ruben lit the way back to the plane with his torch-like flash light. I was glad to get buckled into the seat. There were few words during the three hour flight back to the Paramaribo hangar.

I felt I had failed.

Back to Zimbabwe: It took six weeks between each of our letters, as there was no email at that time, just snail-mail to bag #2034, but I did agree to go to Zimbabwe and help Chamboko set up a program. The Global Health Council estimated 25% sero-prevalence in Zimbabwe. But who really knew because, once again, there was no surveillance data and so many people were dying of diseases that could have been, but were not confirmed, to be caused by AIDS. Malaria and TB were ravishing the country, although there were good medical treatments for these diseases in the capital of Harare. If a person does not respond to the medicine, it *could* indicate an immuno suppression that *could* be due to HIV/AIDS.

I found the money for air fare and training supplies, and—since this would be my first time going to Africa, which made me a bit uneasy—I asked a friend, Duane, an AIDS educator, to come with me for moral support. We arrived in Zimbabwe in October 1999, full of apprehensions, full of unknowns.

The first night we stayed in the town of Chinhoyi at the house of a very friendly couple, Michael and Anneke Schneider. Michael was from Germany, Anneke from The Netherlands, and they were with the German Development Services (GDS), helping with Zimbabwe's transportation needs. In the course of Michael's work, he had met

Chamboko in the small village of Chivende—where Chamboko had been speaking about AIDS prevention—and had offered to help Chamboko with transportation to the bush community, since Chamboko was without a vehicle and Michael had a truck.

I am reminded of a little incident that still makes me smile. Duane and I were to share a room. No problem, I thought, because I didn't know yet that Duane snored like a dragon. As I settled into the shared space, I tore off the baggage tags from the duffle bags and tossed them into a straw basket. Then the basket shimmied so of course I had to look inside. NO exaggeration, well just a bit, there was a huge fuzzy black spider larger than my clinched fist awakened from his little nap before I assaulted him with my trash. I shuddered – I *really, really* intensely dislike and fear spiders, especially the big furry ones. I'm mildly arachnophobic, I'd say.

In an angelic plea, I asked Duane if he could empty the basket with a teeny little spider and toss the little guy into the bush. He heroically said, "No problem!" like he always does when he has a chance to be macho. As Duane picked up the wastebasket, he squealed like a little girl, dancing

179

around in circles. "Ew, ew, ew, that is no teeny spider!" he snarled at me. Yes, the image of Duane running into the bush on his tippy-toes, screaming like a stuck pig honestly makes me giggle as I write this fourteen years later!

There was another incident involving Duane and the indigenous critters of international travel: We were in the Chitwan National Park just outside of Kathmandu, Nepal. Having completed a series of HIV/AIDS prevention trainings with sponsorship from UNESCO, we were awarded two nights off from the big city. Joined by peer trainers Amrit and Renu, Duane and I decided to go for a hike in the Chitwan jungle. We were told to wear long pants and long sleeved shirts because of the predominance of blood sucking slugs that hid in the bush vines. They were horrible little things that landed on your skin looking like a small piece of string and within seconds, when they were engorged with blood, they resembled fat macaronis.

There was a very specific technique for removing the 'macaroni slug' – burn it before his head burrowed deeply into the skin. Duane's lit cigarette and lighter were used for the demise of the blood suckers, and we continued our jungle trek. It was not until we returned to the camp that I realized one of those little suckers managed to evade our careful scrutiny. I noticed that my shirt was covered with blood and in a panic, I ripped out the slug from my right breast! In my haste, the head was definitely left in my body. My right boob swelled to orange-size with the infection.

It was not until I returned to the US that I was told that I would forever be reminded of the jungle hike with slugs because I was now infected with a virus that manifested first as a small dermatological itch and later as a deep purple blemish that looked like an intense birth mark. Of course this insult was activated by stress, much like the herpes virus, and most often covered significant portions of my face. It took a panel of four Dermatologists to determine this unfortunate fate.

Oh, the everlasting memories of international escapades. And, once again, I have digressed from my discussion of working in Zimbabwe!

Days after our stay in Chinoyi, we moved to the village of Majunge to lodge at an absolutely horrible 'motel'. I know that sounds very judgmental but, from my perspective, that's the way it really was. The rooms were filthy, the wash room had chunks of excrement scattered in front of flooded toilets and the communal shower dripped brown foul smelling water.

That night, after Duane and I had our first experience of eating sadza with our fingers, there were terrible screams in the wash room. Of course I had to get up to see what was going on and if I could help in any way. In the very dim shadow of the motel lamps I witnessed a woman getting brutally raped. This was not a good omen for our stay in Majunge.

In the early morning, Duane and I were up and ready to go, as scheduled by Chamboko the night before. We were anxious to get to our training venue in the bush community of Chivende, a good 250 miles or three hours away. I was told the roads were very rudimentary and primitive, so I wanted to get an early start. The watered-down tea in my plastic mug went from lukewarm to Zimbabwean ambient temperature as we sat on broken wooden benches in front of the motel.

One hour went by and then the second. In the third

hour, we sighted Chamboko in a cloud of red dust driving a sputtering white pickup truck. "Terrific," we thought, now we can start the journey to waiting students and teachers. But – almost expected – there was yet another glitch before our departure. Chamboko explained that we would first take a quick detour to the medical clinic in the small town of Karoi to meet with administrators who had the funds for our program.

We went to the hospital, and we waited, and waited, and waited. Clearly, patience is not one of my virtues. It was really frustrating for me to sit and waste time like this. Chamboko kept coming back to us saying that the woman who would disburse the money is with someone else but we'll get the money today. We waited some more. I was fit to be tied while Duane more maturely told me to 'chill out'. Easier said than done, I thought, acknowledging in a grump that I was a type A-plus personality. When time rolled around to three in the afternoon, however, I knew there was no money. Chamboko emerged from closed doors just shaking his head, grumbling, "There is no funding, only a little bit for petrol." My heart sank.

To make matters worse, our plan had been to arrive at

Chivende in the early morning to take part in a big welcoming ceremony to meet the villagers, training participants and most importantly, the Chief and his Council. It was the first time Americans and white folks had been invited to the school, so there was great excitement and preparation. Apparently they wouldn't believe that we were actually coming until they saw us in person. But we still were not there. And there were no telephones to let them know we were disastrously late. Fuming and admittedly being a big baby, I followed Duane into the truck and remained silent for the first two hours of travel to Chivende.

When we drove into the school at six that evening, there were only seven people – the others had left. Juliet and Tawanda, the student coordinators, almost bowled us over with their enthusiastic hugs. Because it was so late and we were told that it was very dangerous to drive 'white people' in the dark, we could only spend about an hour talking with the villagers. They kept saying, "We didn't think you were coming." Of course, the chief and the traditional healers had left already, since they'd waited all day for us. We drove back to Majunge to pack up all of our posters, training materials and clothes. Early the next day we left for a six day assignment in Chivende.

I don't really know what Chamboko did with most of the money he got for transportation, because there were only vapors of petrol to do any outreach to the neighboring schools. There were rumors that Chamboko had a girl friend in Karoi and used our precious fuel to visit her daily. He'd say, "We can't do the events today, because we have an empty tank," and then I'd have to donate some of my own money to buy gas to get to where we were going.

One time we were driving to get some gas an hour's drive from Chivende. I was a passenger because I had the money! The journey was on an incredibly rocky, rutted road where we used a high volume of our precious gas avoiding the boulders and fallen rocks. Chamboko murmured that he had a good idea: he would to save petrol by turning off the ignition while we were going down a hill. Duane quickly cautioned him, "Please don't cut the engine because you will lose control of the driving mechanism," but Chamboko retorted, "I want to save gas!"

Sure enough he did exactly that—turned off the

motor, the steering locked up and we drove right into a deep ditch. After finally rescuing the car, I recommended that Chamboko please let Duane drive. The two hour delay got us back to Chivende well into the night.

Our botched funding in Zimbabwe was only one of several financial fiascos that I experienced internationally. I was promised by hosting organizations that there was financial support. Hence, I arrived with three big bags full of training materials, presents, manuals and posters, and— guess what?—my host had no money to conduct the trainings. With Chamboko there finally were some harsh words, because I couldn't rely on him at all.

Anyway, one afternoon, before we'd started the trainings, Chamboko and I were walking around mud huts in Chivende, and little kids would see me and yell, "Muzungu, Muzungu!" Then all you could hear was a rustling of bushes and peals of laughter coming from hidden children. I had no idea what was going on but still the shuffling of leaves and giggles.

Then, once again, "Muzungu, Muzungu," and I looked at Chamboko and asked, "Who are they calling Muzungu

186

and what does Muzungu mean?" Chamboko, kind of embarrassed, said, "That's you—it means 'white person'. That's what they call white people here in Zimbabwe: Muzungu." Thereafter, I had the nick name 'Muzungu Wendy'. It didn't seem like any of these kids had ever seen a white person before because they just stared. It was a real novelty for them to see someone who wasn't black.

So, no matter where I went, the kids would always shout, "Muzungu, Muzungu Wendy!" When I approached little babies to comment on how adorable they were, they would wrinkle their noses into a knot and then start screaming, because they were so scared. "Hello, cutie, mhoro, mhoro" or "ossibye otiano," which are greetings that would hopefully calm them, but they returned the favor with wailing and would hide behind whatever gave them a supposed distance from me. I finally discovered that this intense fear was because their parents had told them that white people eat black African babies. There I was, 'the white devil.'

There was more of an acceptance of white people in the city of Harare, the capital of Zimbabwe, but certainly not here, about two hundred and fifty miles out, in the bush of Chivende and Majunge. This may have had to do with the culture of witchcraft where the curses and stories were passed on from generation to generation. It was like our concept of a boogey man.

When we conducted our educational sessions in Chivende, it was terribly dry and the red dust literally stuck to your teeth. I was outrageously thirsty and there was minimal precious bottled water. We begged one of the Chivende school teachers, Jonga, to drive his motorcycle to Karoi for water. When we were this parched, we would pay anything for water. We were supposed to start the training at ten, which, I discovered, in Africa means people get there at twelve or one, even if they live around the corner. Yet, many of the students actually had to walk 5-10 miles to attend school. The cemented class room had no ventilation and it was very dark, seemingly to insulate us from the hot African sun. Forty kids finally showed up, all lined up at their school desks. I only knew a few words of their language, but there was a man named Willard who was there to translate from Shona, the native tongue of Zimbabwe, a really lovely language.

During the training, there were some wonderful ladies

who helped with the cooking for the participants. There were four of them—I just called them 'mummies'—and the best way to describe them is 'adorable'! They prepared sadza and cassava, the corn meal staple food with a mashed potato consistency. Along with beans, we would slurp up the sadza with our fingers. Sometimes we had treats of chicken heads or chicken feet to augment the bland sadza. All of this was prepared in a big blackened pot over an open fire just outside of the medical clinic where we slept.

With these mummies was a very very shy woman by the name of Consuelo, around thirty years old, who huddled pensively in the corner of an area used for food preparation. She was silent as others bustled chopping leaves and potatoes. I tried to engage her with light conversation, but she returned my attempts with blank stares. After two days, Willard came over to me and whispered, "Her name is Consuelo. She has AIDS. She wants to talk with you and share her feelings as she asks some questions."

I said I'd love to meet with her, so during one of the lunch breaks I met with Consuelo and Willard where we sat on a straw woven mat in one of the clinic rooms and closed the door. When I introduced myself, speaking very slowly for Willard's interpretation, Consuelo's head and eyes were focused downwards to the mat. I could see how broken and rejected she felt.

She had visibly swollen glands, lung problems, very deformed feet and it was clear that she was in tremendous pain. She explained she was very concerned about her two children, who were in another village, and told me how hopeless and helpless she felt, having this disease called 'Slim'. 'Slim' was the name she knew for AIDS, a word describing the emaciation notoriously associated having HIV/AIDS. Another name in Africa for the acronym AIDS, not known to Consuelo, was 'the American Invention to Discourage Sex'!

I tried to comfort her by saying, "I can see how very sad you are, but there is a lot of hope—I have friends all over the world who've been living with AIDS for many many years," but nothing I said seemed to help. I finally asked her to tell me about something that made her happy, but she replied "Nothing makes me happy." So, then I said, "Tell me about what you *used* to like to do—maybe something when you were young." She replied, "I used to like to sew with my Aunties and friends in school. I responded, "Wonderful! And what kinds of clothes did you make?" I really wanted to keep the conversation positive and flowing.

Now there was a little more eye contact as she told me, "We liked to get together in the afternoons and we would make little blouses and skirts." Then with a shy smile and upward glance, she added, "and we talked about the boys in the school." Gently, I kept prodding her on, "Tell me more about the boys and about the sewing."

The more she talked about the memories, the more she began to straighten up. She was looking at me, smiling with new encouragement. At least she had something upbeat to think about, even though it was only a memory. But she was more animated and even giggled a bit.

I had to get back to the training and was disappointed to see that when I left her with the other mummies in the kitchen she was once again crawling into her corner, pulling down her little woolen hat so no one could see her eyes.

When I returned to the teenagers, I said, "I just met the most wonderful person! She lives with AIDS and she's right here in your own village. In our conversation, she said she'd be willing to share her story with all of us."

This would also give me an opportunity to talk about the importance of 'confidentiality' when discussing the lives of our friends with HIV/AIDS. I'd encouraged Consuelo to come and speak with the youth, with the offer of a little present, and hoped that her words would give the peer educators more of a commitment to our program and a reality of the epidemic. It would be beneficial to let them know that HIV/AIDS *is right here* among them and isn't always someone else's problem. I also explained to them that Consuelo used to like to sew and maybe we could get some material for her, so she could keep happily busy.

So, after the training that afternoon, four of us went to the little supply store in town, a place that had only minimal types of items, but there was one piece of material, which we bought, along with two needles and a spool of thread. We invited Consuelo to come to our training the next morning where we gave her the material, telling her, "We want you to make whatever you want!"

She just beamed and giggled as she massaged the green printed cloth. "I haven't had a needle in my hand so long, I don't know if I can do it," she explained in her dialect of Shona, but I told her, "Well, we'll be there to help you if you need it."

For the next three days I could see her, still at her little spot in the kitchen, sewing but now she was interacting and conversing with others. We were only going to be there for another two days and now noticed that she included the other mummies with her needle work – she seemed to be rushing now. I was delighted to see that it was clear she enjoyed the company of the young students and was having her meals with us. She just didn't seem to focus so much on the AIDS now.

Then, the last day we were there, she handed me the skirt she'd been working on. She had made the lovely skirt for me and to this day I have that Zimbabwean treasure! I take the skirt with me when I do the trainings in Africa and I tell that story to let them know there's always something we can do for a person living with AIDS.

I've done this interactive listening in other places. I try

to get people living with HIV/AIDS to think about something optimistic and it actually seems to have a physical effect on them. It's like a personal enlightenment of hope, because when I first met Consuelo, she was sullen, complaining, coughing and holding her aching chest. Then, when she was sewing she wasn't talking about her physical problems and was smiling. I did hear that Consuelo died a year later.

Duane and I stayed two weeks on that first trip to Africa. We trained the trainers in Mugunje for five days, we trained the youth peer educators in Chivende, and we also did outreach presentations in local schools in other communities, briefly, with translators. I afterwards lost touch with the people there because the political situation in Zimbabwe became extremely dangerous. Regretfully, we have since heard that several of the youth peer educators and outreach volunteers were murdered by the revolutionaries.

I want to share one more memory of the 'power of positive thinking'. I am reminded of a lovely woman who did counseling of Cameroonians who test positive at the Limbe Hospital. Juliet was a participant at one of our

"Train the Trainers" workshop in Mutengene. We were hosted by the Baptist Convention and Melvine Wajiri had done miraculous work finding local sponsors for our activities. Actually, Melvine was an exemplary international associate because of this demonstrated attribute in confirming five sponsoring agencies for the HIV/AIDS prevention through peer education trainings in Cameroon. They superbly provided transportation, meals for the participants, my accommodations with nine others in a guest house, and bottled water, always a precious commodity.

Juliet pulled me aside during one of our breaks. She described that she could actually feel the AIDS virus multiplying and moving through her body. She shivered, rubbing her arms as she explained the vibrations and chills that were supposedly caused by HIV. This was not new to me – psychosomaticism: your mind plays very vivid and physical games when you believe what others are saying. I think this is also called the 'medical student syndrome' where students actually manifest the symptoms that *could* occur with various maladies. Sometimes it's better not to read possible side effects when purchasing a medicine!

As Juliet continued to tremble, mimicking one trying to get warm, I decided that I would extend the psycho-somaticism concept a little longer. I told her I had a very special and magical bracelet that would make her feel better. I was careful not to give her false hope. My gift was a personalized PWA bracelet that I had ordered for the family and close friends of Mark Bard, who died of AIDS on May 2, 1991. His death is still a painful memory for me. It was called a PWA bracelet because it was manufactured only for "People With AIDS" or their immediate families. I ordered twenty and brought one to Cameroon with the hope of giving it to an African in need of moral support.

She put the silver bracelet on her right hand. I noticed how frightfully thin she was as I bent the circular ornament to her miniscule size. I explained that if she held the metal, particularly if she was sad, it would get increasing warm and this warmth would fight the HIV and make her happy. Now this wasn't a total lie because the warmth from her hand would be transferred to the metal giving her the heat sensation. I was hoping for the power of positive thinking.

When Juliet returned to the training the following day,

she jubilantly came up to me exclaiming, "It worked, the magic bracelet worked! I held tightly onto it and the HIV has stopped moving in my body!" For the next several days I would glance over to Juliet to see her massaging Mark's bracelet with her other hand. She was clearly more optimistic and happy now. Was this Mark continuing to share his love?

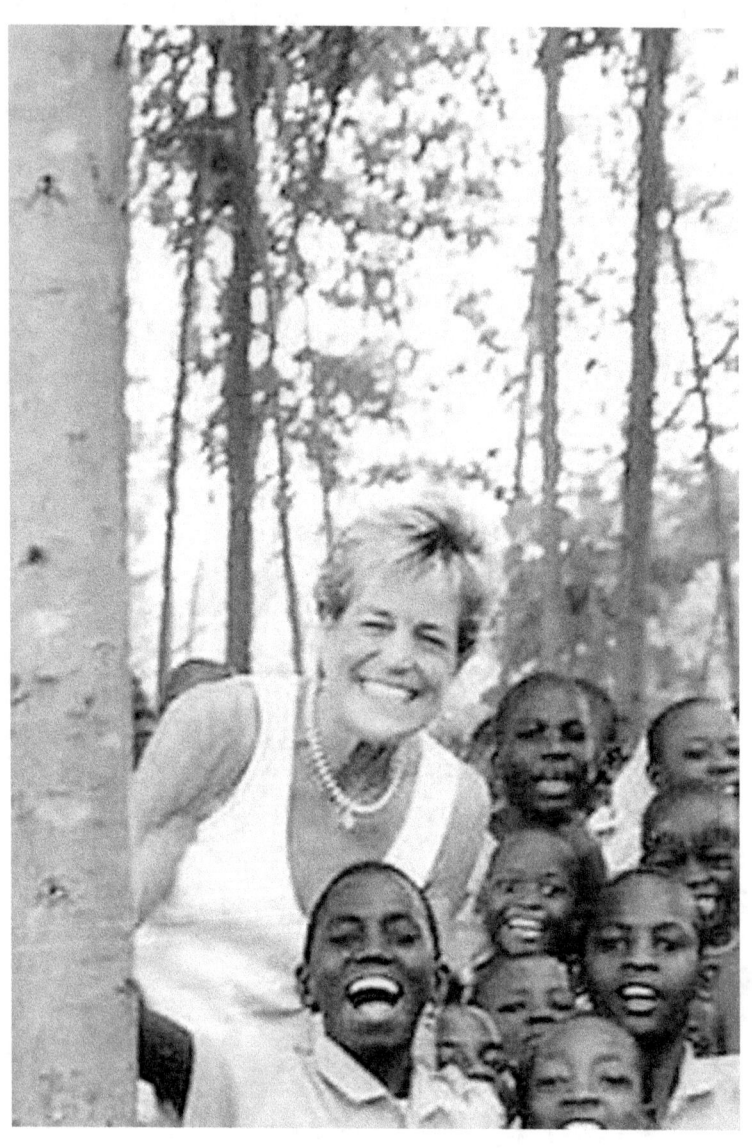

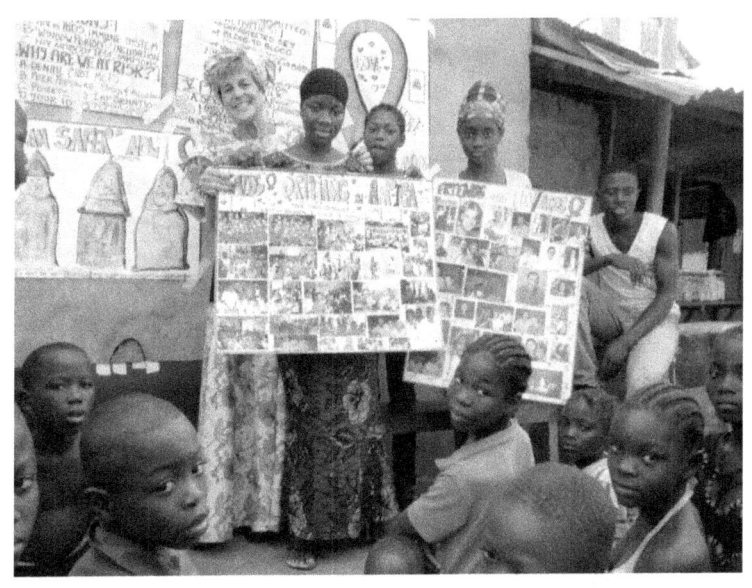

Outreach into the slums of Monrovia, Liberia

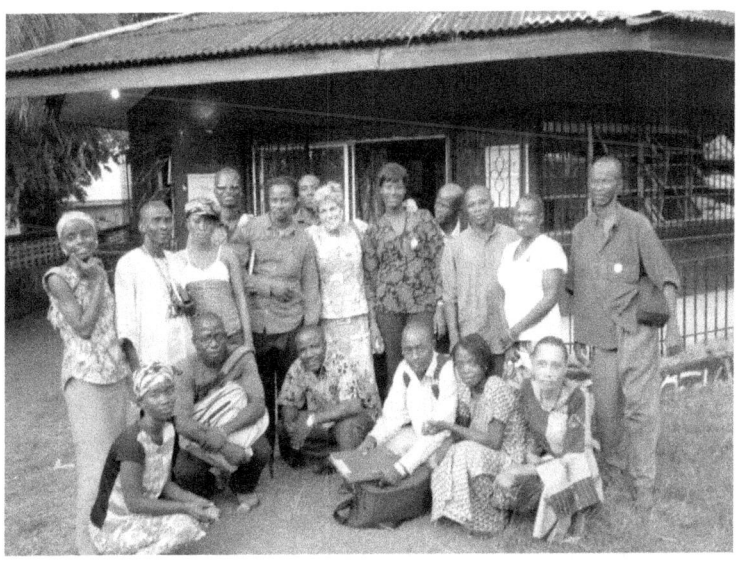

Liberians living with HIV/AIDS in the Light Foundation

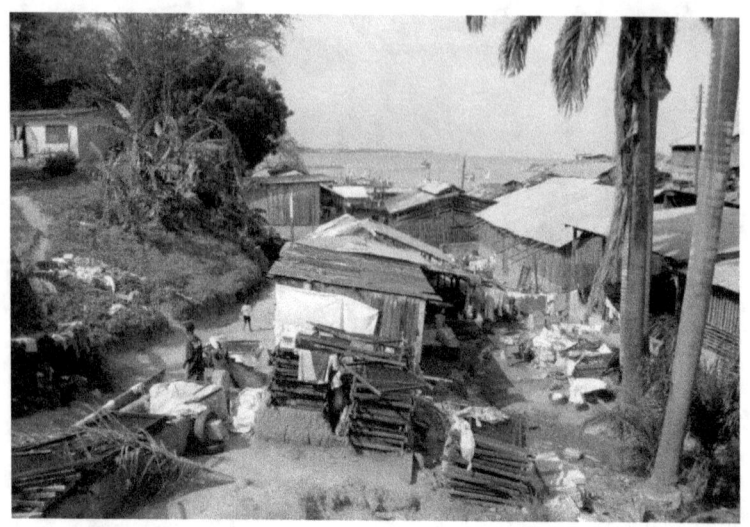

Takoradi fishing village at our training site for the Ghanaian military

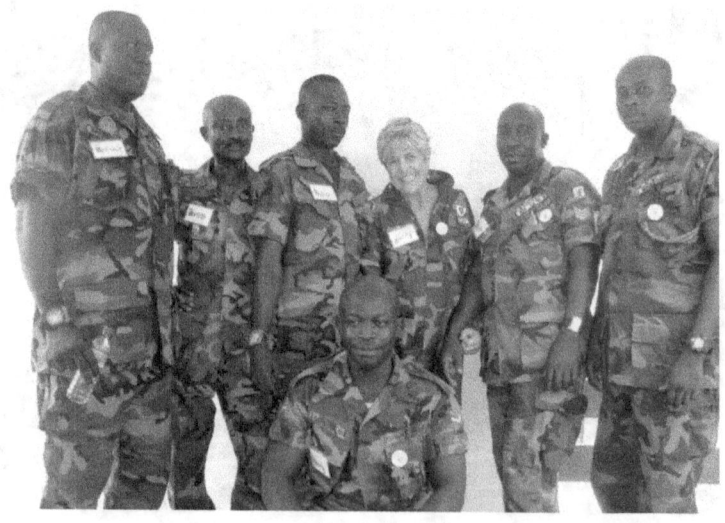

Peer education with the military in Takoradi, Ghana

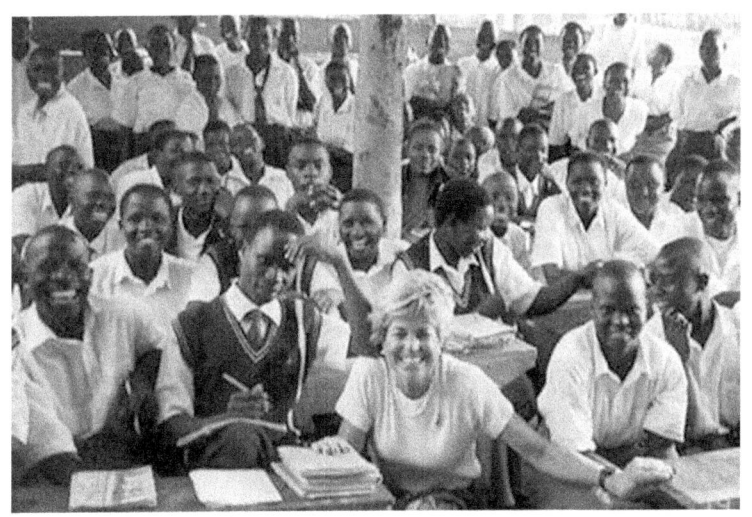

Light High School, Kayunga, Uganda

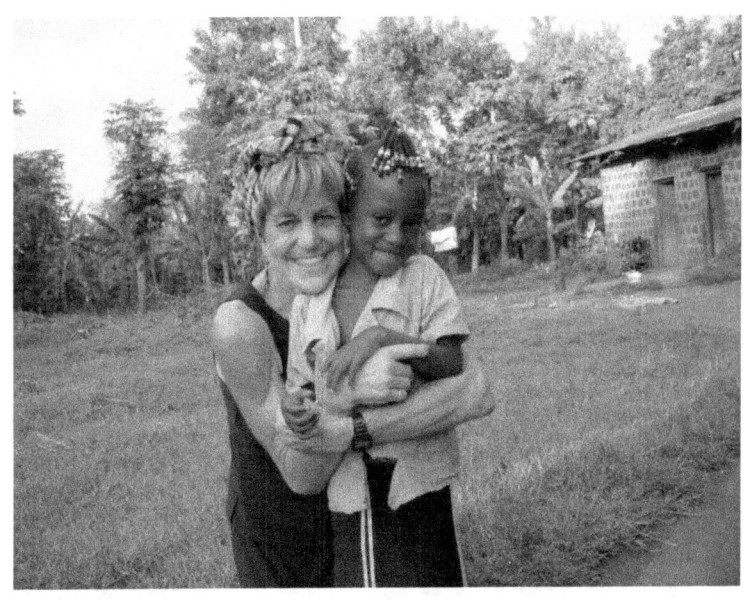

Baby Wendy

201

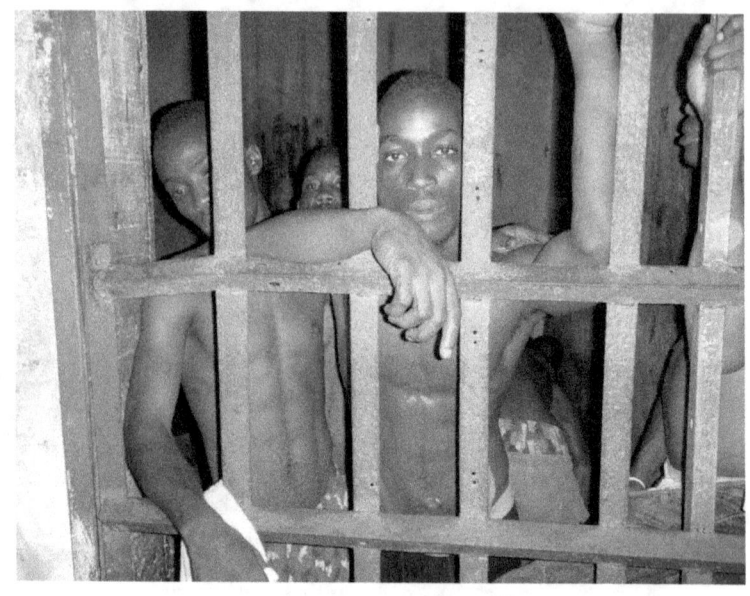

Liberia prison

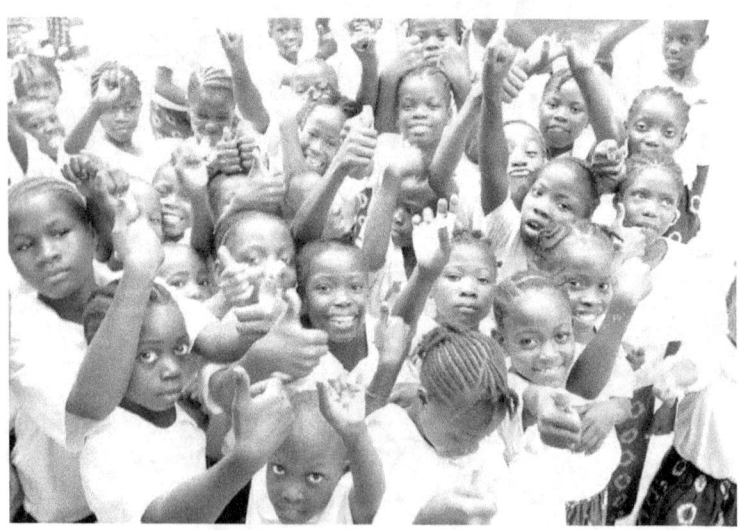

Obass girls with my nail polished thumbs

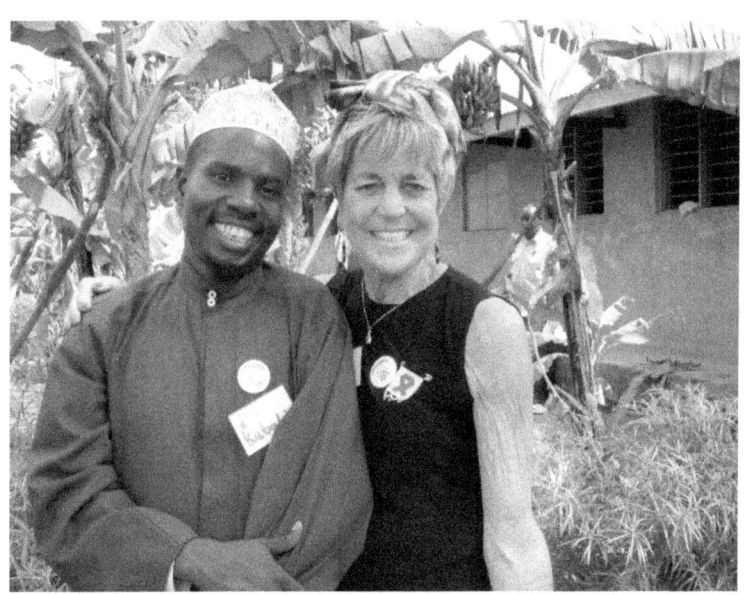

Sheikh Kabali Idris, Uganda

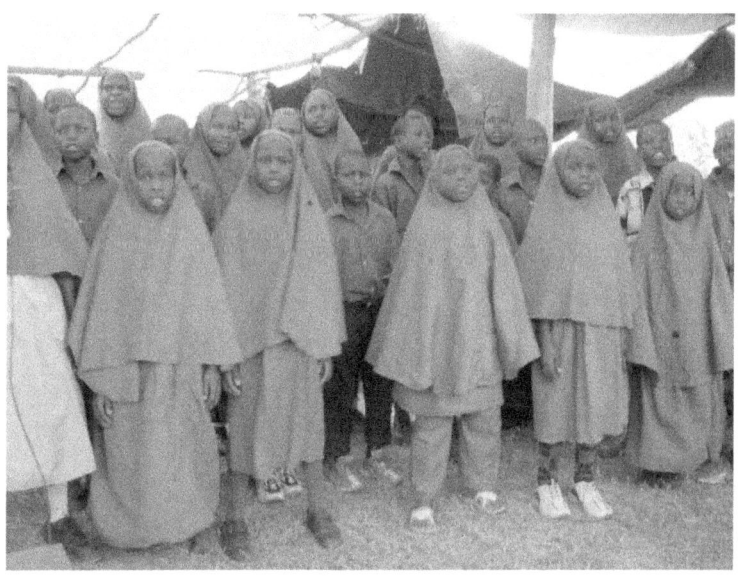

Islam community, Uganda

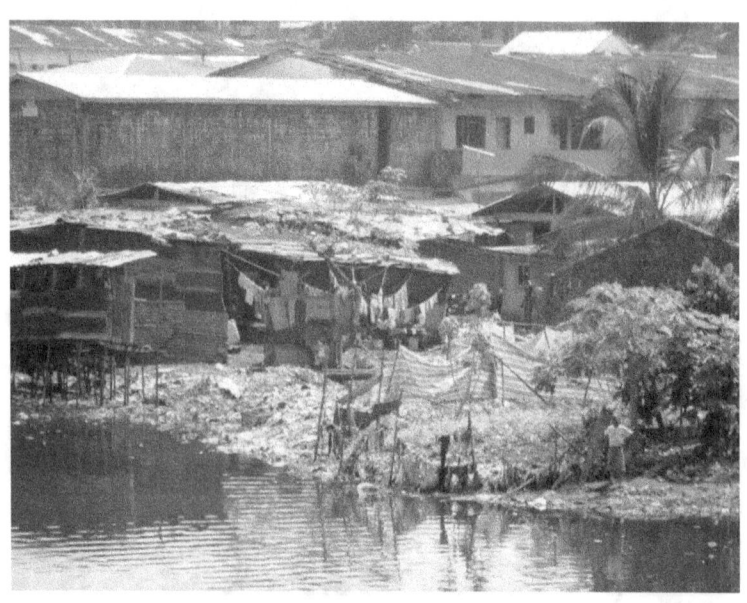

The slums of Monrovia, Liberia

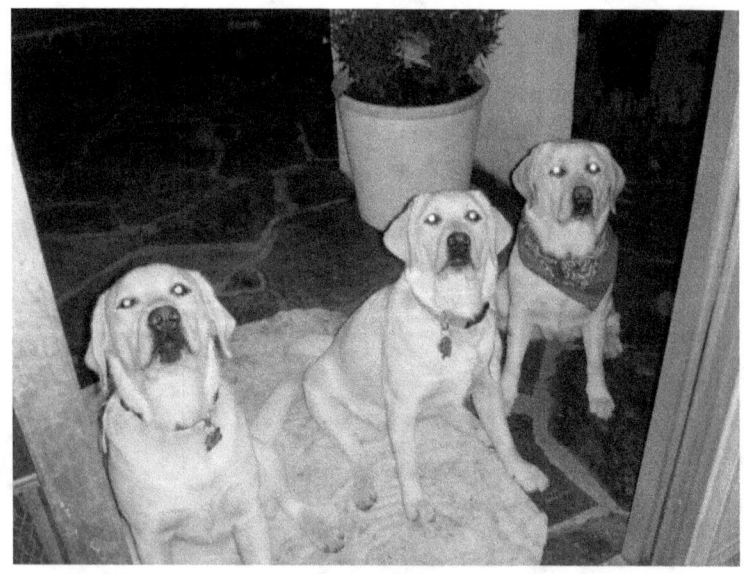

Eupe, Kinshasa, Muzungu

Uganda

I was in Africa again, January, 2000, this time by myself, coming off the airplane in Kampala, Uganda. The man who sponsored the trip was the Rev. Fred Taabu, from the Kampala Baptist Union. I got off the plane, with all of my bags, very anxious to meet him. "That must be the Reverend", I surmised, as I saw a black man with a big sign that said "Wendy". I'd learned some Lugandan phrases and I went running over to him and his colleagues, and I gave him a big hug, which he just loved, because here was a white person, coming from a foreign land, giving him a hug, and he was so excited about this.

However, the excitement and the thrill quickly turned into a feeling of despair, because Rev. Taabu now said, "Well, we prayed to the Lord Jesus Christ for funding, but, alas, we didn't get it," although he'd told me there was solid funding to do the programs, the trainings, for both the teenagers and the trainers. So I rather awkwardly blurted out, "Reverend Fred, you pray to the Lord Jesus Christ for guidance, for strength, for courage to find resources—you don't pray for money to drop into your hands."

But all he could say was, "We have no money."

"What does that mean—what do we do?" I responded.

"I don't know," he told me.

Oh my, I was reliving the Zimbabwean nightmare of zero funding for any activities, not even accommodations. It was very hot and muggy, I was dead tired and my senses were numb from 46 hours of traveling. Finally the Rev. Taabu said he had a friend who ran a Congolese hostel outside of the city of Kampala. I was making no sense and blindly went along with the plan.

So we lugged my bags to the bustling bus station and piled into a mutate—a Volkswagen-sized van already teeming with late night travelers. Now, taking any public transportation in Kampala is a nightmare, and then here's this white meat, and everyone is saying, "Muzungu, Muzungu." And they're all trying to touch me, and it's late, and I'm tired, and we have no money, and I just couldn't be more frustrated or exhausted.

What was I going to do for three weeks in Uganda without any money? A plane wasn't even going to leave for two weeks, but then I decided come hell and high water I was going to figure out a way to do the trainings.

So we went to the Congolese hostel of Rev. Fred's friend, Mr. Pascal, just outside of Kampala, with all my bags. The place smelled of urine and rat feces. There were about a dozen people staying there, a motley crew, to say the least, no other whites but me. On this first trip to Uganda, I don't remember seeing any whites at all, until I got back to Kampala for my flight home.

They took me into a very small private room—walls made of some sort of peeling concrete, windows with fixed bars but no glass, screens with huge holes in them, so I knew the bugs were going to be in there with me that night. I could see smashed bugs on the walls, which other guests had killed—big wasp-type mosquitoes and other insects, and anything with more than four legs I don't like.

There was a small hole in the concrete floor of my

room that served as a latrine—terrible stench, teeming with bugs inside it. Next to that there was just a pipe with a trickle of water, which was supposed to be for washing, but we would instead get a couple of buckets full of dirty river water and bathe with that. Bed was just a woven mat on the ground.

That first night, I was totally miserable. I hadn't eaten yet, so I looked into the kitchen of the hostel, and there was just this tiny little man, Mr. Abdul, who spoke French, since the Congolese speak French. Good! I would be able to communicate with him, but my enthusiasm was quickly tempered when I saw what he was preparing. It was rice, out of which he was picking bugs, and there were rancid tomatoes bursting with big white worms. I thought, "Good thing I brought my own food." I always bring a little stash of tuna fish, squirtable mayonnaise, wheat thins, cheese, power bars—the essentials. So that night I made myself a mixture of a power bar, tuna fish, and mayonnaise, finally curled up on the mat, and, since there were no sheets, took some clothes from my bag and put them around me.

Then the mosquitoes came. *Big* mosquitoes—big, buzzzzzz, mosquitoes. So, I'd get up, get my flashlight, try to find out where they were, try to swat them, get back on my mat—it happened over and over again, hour after hour. I now had my pants on my head, and that was hot, so I was sweating and couldn't breathe. Well, the mosquitoes were really getting to me physically and emotionally and I could feel the bugs crawling all over me, but I was dealing with the insect stuff.

Next the rats arrived. I heard the scratching of ugly toenails across the dirt and turned on my flashlight to see about a dozen big rats, just sauntering idiotically around. They were used to people, because when Abdul in the kitchen would see them, he would just kick them away, they'd come back, and he'd boot them off again. He didn't kill them or hurt them, just knock them away. There was garbage everywhere in the kitchen so they would ramble back in.

Since a religious group was sponsoring me and I really needed some humor at this moment, I named the rats after the twelve disciples, then shooed them away. But the biggest one always came back. I heard this "crunch, crunch, crunch," and it was the same old fat guy, who I'd named Judas. Well, Judas had gotten into my green duffle bag, into my wheat thins. That's when I lost my sense of humor. I was ticked off. Nobody gets into my precious wheat thins! I said to Judas rat, "Now you are in big trouble!"

I picked up my sneaker and humanely whapped him on his butt. He hardly took notice and continued munching. The whaps increased in intensity and number but he kept coming back. This 'game' continued for about fifteen aggravating minutes. This was *not* funny. Then I had an idea. One of my L.A.P.D. cop friends had given me, for an emergency, a little can of Mace, so I found it and went after Judas. I said, "Judas, you're going to die." I squirted him in his face, and he just looked at me and twitched his nose—didn't react at all. So, I said, "Oh, yeah, you think I'm done?" And then I squirted him about ten more times with the Mace.

By this time I was almost maniacal, but Judas wasn't bothered at all, just started sauntering off. *I* was asphyxiated—I couldn't breathe—my eyes were tearing, I felt nauseous, I needed air. So, at three o'clock in the morning, I went, with my pants still around my head, with whatever clothing I could find, out into the bush, curled up into a ball—and cried. I just cried....

The next morning I had a meeting with the people from the Kampala Baptist Union. I was particularly impressed with the director, Mr. Alex Wanyama, who was clearly chagrined with the situation of the promised funding. In a convincing tone, he reprimanded the Reverend Tabbu explaining to him, "What you did is unethical—inviting Wendy to Uganda, telling her she would have money, and then having no money for her trainings."

He sympathetically looked over at me and offered, "We will see if we can go to one of the churches and talk with some of the teenagers at the church groups." And that's exactly what we did. We found 40 young church goers at the Baptist Church in Kyebando who were the first peer educators with PEP/Uganda. We still had no money for the food, so I bought beans and rice for the kids for the four days of training.

The students ranged in age from 12 to 24 years. Most came from the tiny village of Kayoye and spoke only Lugandan. I had no interpreter, so pretty much acted our mission of HIV/AIDS prevention and the need to stop

211

discrimination of Ugandans living with the disease. It's funny how much can be communicated with hands and body language! Most of the students were orphans to AIDS and had lost their entire families. I showed them my posters with pictures of my friends who were living with HIV/AIDS or who had died. They thought that AIDS was only in Africa, not in the Western world. I told stories of my friends, and we formed a bond of mutual empathy.

Many shared experiences of how their parents got sick and died in total isolation. Several went to live with aunts and uncles, but they died too. The family unit could be twenty members with the thirteen-year-olds as the oldest and the ones responsible for the others. There was no information about AIDS, and they were desperately afraid because no one knew how the 'sickness' went through the village so rapidly. They were told that it was a curse for people who did not believe in God. It was witchcraft for those who sinned. One got sick being in the same hut or school with one with this curse. There was nothing to do; AIDS was a fate.

After gaining their trust and understanding that I was

trying to help the community, I described that the disease was totally preventable. There were specific behaviors associated with AIDS and these behaviors could be avoided. We talked about a little germ, like a little bug, yes, it was the virus that goes from one person to another. Then we discussed the dangers of blood-to-blood activities like the sharing of knives for ceremonial tribal markings. Next we talked about little babies getting the virus of AIDS, HIV, from their infected mummies.

Finally, we carefully broached the subject of sex. I explained that embarrassment and feeling uncomfortable was OK because sex was something they all *did,* but never talked about. They all knew what it was but didn't know what it was called. "Why do people have sex?", I queried. "People have sex to make babies and to make money," they replied. But it was made very clear to me by the Baptist Union that I could not talk about condoms in this church. I asked Reverend Fred, "How do you want me to talk about prevention?" And he said, "Abstinence, just abstinence," so that's what I did.

But at the breaks, some kids who could speak a little English were telling me, "We all have sugar daddies, we've been having sex since we were eight years old. What's all this about abstinence? Where will I get my school fees—I need to do sex for my school fees—where do you think I got my shoes? If we didn't have sugar daddies or sugar mommies, we wouldn't have clothes. Where do you think I get my food, where do you think my mother gets her food?" So they told me about being sold for sex.

Then I'd ask the kids, "Well, if you knew of people who were having sex, what would you recommend they do?" Of course they'd say use condoms, so I hadn't said the word to be in compliance with Rev. Fred, but during the breaks when the kids were telling me about how much sex they were having, they'd ask, "Where do we get these condoms?" If the Rev. came in to the classroom, there would be a big hush, but, fortunately, he wasn't there for much of the training, so we could talk informally about condoms, which were available in some of the local clinics.

I had a favorite student, a little girl named Prossy, only twelve and one of the stars in our training. Prossy asked me to go to her village and meet her family. She said the village was very close, so we trekked over this tiny path and finally reached her community, an hour and a half later. Everyone knew that Muzungu was coming, so they did a special dance for me and offered me food. God only knows what it was but it was terribly salty.

In Prossy's village, there wasn't anyone over the age of fifteen. There were no adults. There were only kids, about three hundred of them. Everyone else in the village had died from AIDS. Prossy told me, "The older people all died. We don't know why, but they died."

Prossy and I formed a special bond and kept in touch first by letters and eventually by emails. When Prossy got married in 2013, she asked me to be her matron of honor. She will always be a friend.

Since we'd done pretty well with the first training for teens at the church in Kyebando, I then moved with Denis Mukiyeye, one of the Congolese guests at Pascal's hostel, by taxi, with all my bags, on rutted and almost impassable roads, to the small village of Kayunga. Many times we had to get out of the old car to push through unbroken passages. Still with no money from the Baptist Union, I was to conduct a 'Train the Trainers' program, for counselors, community outreach workers and directors of NGOs. That experience in Uganda was a turning point for me, because I was *living* with Ugandans, in the bush, away from the big city of Kampala. There was no running water or electricity as nine of us sat in the dark on broken concrete in a medical clinic.

Often I would get them laughing and could follow the strikingly white teeth from one side of the room to the other. Eventually we combined our resources and found some candles – mine! In the morning, Pastor Harrison found some kids to pick mangoes for our breakfast. Meeting these minor challenges brought us very close together. This was a very precious experience for me.

I usually held the trainings with the adults from nine to three, then had the rest of the afternoon off. In Kayunga, one of our trainers was Moses, who ran the Kisaaba Center for 162 AIDS orphans. Moses knew that I loved walking and exploring the villages so we met after the training for our daily adventure. In these bush communities, everyone knew Moses and he knew everyone! Moses loved introducing me to his friends and parading me around like his little trophy.

One time, Moses and I walked through gnarled vines toward an opening where there were five little mud huts. We heard shrills of "Jambo, jambo" and "Oli otya" from a group of twelve children all under age 11 years. Walking up to a lovely woman holding a brand new baby we were greeted with smiles of recognition for Moses. Victoria showed us her newborn girl and asked us for a nice Christian name for the infant. Moses exclaimed, "Wendy!" I wrote the name in the red dirt and Victoria seemed pleased with the choice. We now had a 'Baby Wendy'. For the next six trips to Kayunga, I brought little dresses, shirts and stuffed animals for 'Baby Wendy'. She is now at Global Junior School where I very happily have paid her school fees for seven years.

But I kept hearing, "Muzungu, Muzungu." Apparently Moses had taught the villagers to call me "Muzungu Wendy." And the term "Muzungu" stuck. I'm Muzungu Wendy.

*

I kept in touch with Prossy and Richard Kintu from the first training in 2000. Through broken English, Richard told me that because he was inspired with our PEP/Uganda training; he told me that he was doing AIDS prevention work at his school. When I was invited back to do a training in Uganda in 2002, I delighted to find that Richard would help me with the educational workshops. I paid for his transportation to and from Makerere University in Kampala. This was a small price to pay for his wisdom.

He's my hero. He's going to make it. This guy is brilliant. He was with me the entire time in 2002. He was one of the oldest in the church groups, about twenty-two then. He was instrumental in the success of the program that year because his specific assignment was not only to help me with translating English into Ugandan, but he would talk to the Ugandan youth about why they were particularly at risk for HIV.

That was so important, because for me to say, "There's a high prevalence of prostitution, promiscuity, and poverty, which often leads to risk-taking behavior." For me to detail these activities would seem like I'm talking negatively and judgmentally about them, that I'm saying

218

it's their fault that they are living with HIV/AIDS. But when *he* said things like, "Ugandan men are raping eight-year-olds," or say, "There's absolutely no education in the schools about any of these issues around health and sexuality," it was far better coming from him than from me.

Richard described how young Ugandan students went to 'sugar daddies' and 'sugar mummies' in exchange for sexual favors to pay for school fees and cell phones. He described that young mothers actively sought sexual partners to pay for food for their babies. He mentioned some cultural reasons that predisposed Ugandans to HIV, such as polygamy and the practice of female genital mutilation where a young girl was taken from primary schools to be 'cut' in the jungles.

Richard shared his personal experience of a group circumcision with ten fifteen year old boys and only one razor available for the removal of the foreskin. And then the tradition of wife inheritance forced the wife of a deceased man to become the sexual property of all of her husband's brothers. Richard was *very* valuable and a lot of fun to be with.

That is the concept of peer education. Peer education is not only effective because of similarities of age and gender, but also because of similarities of experience and identification. There is no 'blame factor.' It's the same with the PEP/LA peer educators—if I say to teenagers, "*You* are at risk because *you* gave in to peer pressure and *you* do dumb things when you're drunk," these phrases are rejected but when a teenager says, "*We* can get pretty stupid when *we* drink and use drugs at our parties," that's a whole lot more effective and credible for the youth at hand.

On this second trip to Uganda, one of the pastors, Harrison, had worked very hard soliciting funds from local sponsors for the series of workshops in HIV/AIDS education through peer education.

Now, one of the greatest expenses of the international projects is petrol for the local transportation. How are you going to get from one village to another? Unless you walk. Well, when these places are three hours by car, over terribly rutted and rocky roads. However, Harrison resourcefully got a financial commitment of $600 from the Kajunga District Council. This was to cover the entire two and a half weeks of training, including the local transportation to far-off villages.

I had told them in the planning stages that my stipulations were, "I will find funding for the international air fare and bring the training materials, but it is the responsibility of the hosting organizations to find local support for accommodations, meals for the participants and a training venue." I feel that this helps to insure involvement of the community members and encourages program sustainability. The District Council of Kajunga allocated some of these funds to each community and each sub-district had to take care of four days of food for their respective participants.

My friend, Shiekh Kabali Idris, was to meet me in the center of Kayunga. Kabali was one of the trainers from the workshops in 2000 and was now the director of YOPDIDA, an organization for disabled Ugandans. With my posters and materials strapped to our backs, we waited for a motorcycle on the dusty road that would take us to Busaana. The image of our scooter chugging and sputtering along at five miles an hour had both of us in stitches! I always have a lot of fun with Kabali.

221

We arrived at the isolated church at 8 a.m. to welcome the forty youth religious leaders. There was nobody there. In fact, three hours later there were still no kids. Eventually we discovered that the people who were to disburse the funds for the training had pocketed the money themselves. No youth, no training venue and no food.

Undaunted, Kabali and I walked around the small village and recruited every young person we could find! It was now 1:30 in the afternoon so I went with three of the Busaana residents to buy food for our now forty participants. I found those tiny sweet bananas and five loaves of very old bread. For the next three hours, we ate and talked at our new training site – the shade of a huge tree. Our group was sustained for three days, and perhaps the inauspicious beginning was a reason for our friendship and success.

After Busaana, we were to try our luck with the sub-district of Galiraya. This time we had a vehicle because the village was four hours by car. There were no sidewalks, of course, so people walked in the middle of the road with their livestock, carts of building supplies and roughly assembled produce. We inched our way through one township, carefully avoiding goats and school children dressed in their brightly colored uniforms. The oncoming assault of logging trucks and fuel tanks was intimidating, as was the helter-skelter of very young children.

We finally arrived at the village of Galiraya and scurried in to meet with the local Council. Of course we were late. The sun was very low. I never like being late, but it is the norm in Africa. The training was to be held in a school, a classroom—no lights, totally dark. We decided to wait until morning. After the welcoming comments from the government officials, chief of the village in full costume and a handful of teachers, we piled back in the car to drive all the way back to Kayunga. How I wanted to accept an invitation to stay with a family, but I was told it was not protocol and was discouraged to remain. We arrived into Kayunga after midnight. My back was screaming from all the jolting travel.

In the morning, we were joined by Dr. Patrick, who would help with translations. Even in daylight it was difficult for the volunteers to see my descriptive posters in the dimly lit classroom made of caked mud. We expected 35 students and had made it very clear that the training for peer educators was to start at 10:00 a.m. This would allow time for some of the kids who had to walk for up to five hours to get to this Galiraya school every day. Of course no one showed up at ten, then half a dozen drifted in, then six more, and finally, by three p.m., when I normally would end a day, all thirty were there. The first day of a training is just chaos, always.

At the end of the day, I made it very clear that the training was going to start *on time* the next day, at ten, and I was serious this time! I told them that ten o'clock was ten American time, not one o'clock Ugandan time and if they were fifteen or more minutes late, they'd have to sing a song, or dance, or read a poem. I do this with all the international trainings.

In every country, teenagers react differently to this mandate. Russian kids hate having to sing or dance or recite in front of a group, so they were always on time. Thai kids, on the other hand, loved it. They came late deliberately—with their tambourines and Thai dresses—so they could sing and dance their cultural traditions for the next two hours. In Africa, they do a Gospel song, and everybody starts singing, clapping and dancing. It really helps with relaxing the participants and building a rapport.

For the second day in Galiraya, there were a couple of people who were late, so there was the outpouring of wonderful, foot stomping, Gospel music, which was just fine. Then, at about twelve o'clock, John walked in with his bicycle. I can still see his face: so black, covered with goggles, pouring sweat, with red mud splattered all over his body from all the puddles he'd ridden through.

John came right up to me and just looked at me, and I said, "John, you're late—you're going to have to sing. Or do you have a good excuse?" He kept looking at me, then put his hands on my shoulders and said, "Miss Wendy, I buried my brother today. He died of AIDS last night."

I couldn't move.

I'd been in Uganda on this trip for about nine days and by now I'd seen too much death, despair and sadness. I had tried to keep strong and somewhat in control. I'm pretty good in emergency situations. I'd been to the villages where no one is older than fifteen. Then the woman who had run screaming out of the Kayunga hospital, screaming that her husband had just died from

225

AIDS. "AIDS, AIDS, AIDS", she hysterically sobbed."
Her wails pierced the night, and she continued until I went
to her and just let her hold me. And now John.

When John told us about his brother, I just folded. It
was 'the last straw'. John was my dissolving point. I could
no longer be the martyr. I could not feel my knees and
wanted to crumble. I held a silent gaze with John, then
wrapped him in my arms and cried uncontrollably. I
looked over his shoulder and could now see that all the
peer educators were also crying and openly sniffling.

"This is exactly why we are here," I said in a broken
voice, "It's because of what John has just shared." Then I
asked, "Would anyone else like to share a similar story?"
That opened Pandora's box. Patrick, my beloved Patrick,
my dear friend, Dr. Patrick, who had previously told me,
with little emotion, that his brother had died from AIDS.
Now he was giving all the details of his brother's last days
and crying the entire time. Everybody in the entire group
was weeping, sobbing, as Patrick told his story.

I just held Patrick's hand, and could see the wet
splashes of his tears getting absorbed by the dry mud floor.

He explained, "I was in denial. I knew he was sick. I'm still in denial. I keep thinking I still see him. Even when I put dirt on his face when he lay in his grave, I tried to convince myself that the person there was not my brother." For *two hours* we listened to similar stories.

I remember glancing but trying not to see the faces of the students in that dark and dank classroom. I clutched Patrick's hand, perhaps too tightly, I don't remember. I held onto the wooden desk for support. The air was heavy and stale. The room thick with emotion, and there was a stifled sound from the throat of one of the peer educators, who just couldn't get the next sentence out—like the cry of a dying bird, in the darkness of that room.

I finally told the peer educators, "I've been pretty strong, seeing what I've seen, experiencing what I have, but I've lost it now. Let's take a thirty minute break."

Then I went outside with Patrick and just bawled.

That was a bonding experience. What's important about the PEP/LA approach is that it *is* so emotional, and flexible. It's OK to go off on a tangent like that, or like the dancing. That's OK. If they want to share something personal, that's very welcome. In Israel, I was talking about the Kubler-Ross stages of dying, right after Yitzhak Rabin had been assassinated, and I said, "I'm sure some of you went through these emotions when you heard the news about Yitzhak Rabin," and then they talked about that for the next two hours. It just poured out of them. It is a surreal moment when you talk about anything that personal.

If there are any positive aspects to HIV and AIDS, this is it. Because when you get this close, and you are sharing your heart and soul and spirit with people, there is a *tremendous bond* formed. We're all in this *together*. It is the commonality of experiences. All this can be very positive.

Africa is always a very precious experience for me.

Goma

I can hardly breathe because my nose is stuffed with little flying bugs. I drool as my teeth clench the flashlight held in my teeth, a torch of hope for more insects. The cacophony of crickets, frogs and bush critters cause quite a racket. I'm the only human awake at the Mokoto Monastery on Kivu Lake. I am the only one awake because the twenty-three brothers and two fathers have an 8:00 p.m. curfew. Their first prayers start at 3:30 a.m., then meditation, more prayers and finally a breakfast of bread, bananas and a sweet fruit resembling a pomegranate. I'm on the porch of one of the brick houses, trying to be as quiet as possible so not to wake my five housemates sleeping on canvas cots.

'Desiree' is my favorite brother, and he thoughtfully brings me water, though it is not potable. He also brings supper – usually rice, potatoes, gunky soup, sometimes a spinachy thing, unidentifiable meat and ghastly little fish.

The environment of the monastery is calm, peaceful, tranquil and pious. During the day, the brothers walk quickly and silently between moments of prayers. There is a soft 'swish' from their simple robes. I wonder—how can they pray seven hours a day? About what? For whom? What are they really thinking? Where does this life of asceticism take them? Why have they chosen to be celibate and why do they have no interest in having a family?

Many have been here for ten years or longer and yet look so very young. I love hearing their songs from the little chapel at 7:00 a.m. and again at 7:45 p.m. Yesterday, I snuck up to the chapel to see them in a circle with sparse chairs. I thought my little visit was unnoticed, but when they returned to our little house, Desiree asked me in French why did I not come in. I think they merely sensed that there was an intruder and did not actually see me.

I'm in Goma, North Kivu, the Democratic Republic of the Congo, to set up PEP/Congo-Goma. The Director of the NGO "MIDEFEHOPS" found me through the Internet in March 2006. Interested in my approach of HIV/AIDS prevention through peer education, Isidore KALIMIRA wrote an email of enquiry. I explained that I had another contact with the NGO "AZUR Developpement" in Congo-Brazzaville and I had hoped to come to the Congo.

Like a dummy, I thought the Congo was one country. Both Sylvie NIOMBO in Congo-Brazzaville and Isidore in DRC informed me that they are two independent countries separated by the Congo River. I quickly researched the geographical differences and felt pretty stupid. But now I had to buy a $100 visa to travel between the two Congos!

Goma is desperately poor. Many people go for days without food. Children eat grass and lick plastic bags. The rags they wear are torn and black with dirt. When five year olds walk ten miles to get water, they are regularly raped by the Congolese military. Then they are raped again when they laboriously return with the filled five gallon plastic water container strapped to their tiny backs.

Volcanic eruptions many years ago spewed lava throughout the city and villages. It's so hard to walk over the piles of lava and rocks, even with my thick-soled Nikes. Literally thousands of kids scamper barefoot through the streets searching for bottle caps and playing with old tires. I've found that the average number of children per family is eight to eleven. Many die at birth. The infants are expendable because there can be many more babies for the woman. The babies are often crippled, deformed and grossly disfigured with warped limbs and curled feet. And yet they wiggle and 'worm' along the roads at a faster pace than I can walk.

Our director, Isidore, recruited fifty-eight teachers, health care providers, hospital personnel, nurses and representatives from Congolese NGOs to be part of our four-day training at the Mokoto Monastery. We were isolated from the rest of the community by huge thirty-foot wooden doors. Outside, the children mimicked my introductory songs, like "Row, Row, Row the boat" and "The Hokey Pokey".

Madeleine, in our workshop, was one of the nurses at the 'Goma Hopital Centrale', where she cared for many women living with AIDS. There is no distinction between HIV and AIDS in the Congo, but I was informed that most of her patients were very sick with diverse opportunistic diseases. I knew there were no dangers from HIV/AIDS but I was a bit leery of contagious open skin ulcers, TB and symptomatic pneumonia. I wanted to visit them.

After the second day of our workshop, I felt comfortable with Madeleine, and she knew I would not be a voyeur of the primitive hospital conditions. She knew that I would accept the environment nonjudgmentally, with a caring purpose.

There were twenty women in varying degrees of the progression of AIDS. Some were accompanied by throngs of relatives and others were motionless and left alone on an iron bed with one thin mattress. The room was littered with used gauze pads, filthy water bowls, discarded bits of food, and there was the pervasive smell of sweat, vomit and medicines.

Madeleine had told them the previous day that "Wendy was coming." I guess that gave them something positive to think about because those who could clapped upon my arrival with Joseph, Isidore and Anurite. Goma is within kilometers of Rwanda, so there is the constant sound of gunfire from the guerillas, heard even in the clinic. The Congolese speak Swahili and French. I communicated with the women in French and a smattering of Swahili.

The experience in the hospital was intense. I immediately went up to one of the first creaky beds and crouched beside the patient and openly stroked her hair. There were still misconceptions of HIV transmission by casual contact, and I could see that some of the family members were concerned with my closeness to the woman. Madeleine translated to and from Swahili from my French.

I had some M&Ms and a handful of LA postcards on which I had written little love notes of hope and comfort. Some of the women were so immobile that, with permission from the nurse, I just gently placed the M&M into the mouth and was awarded with a smile. How they loved the morsels of chocolate! I showed photographs of my USA friends living with HIV/AIDS explaining that this disease is throughout the world. They thought it was only in Africa.

Two beds further, Josephine was comatose. Her cousin spooned diluted milk into her mouth with no response. Her tribal markings were deeply engraved in parallel lines just below her prominent cheek bones. She was frightfully emaciated, frail and in a fetal position. Her eyes were glossed and vacant. There was no response when I talked with her, whispering into her right ear. She'd been in a coma for three days, and Madeleine quietly explained that she was close to death. I kissed Josephine's face while explaining that she was a beautiful, and it was OK to let go, to be with God and to join the angels in Heaven. I had done this so many times with my dying friends in Los Angeles.

After more than ten minutes, just stroking her bone-thin arms, I moved on to the next bed. As before, I murmured that they were not alone, they are loved by God and that I am in Goma to share that there is some hope. Was there? I so believe in the power of positive thinking.

Twenty minutes after I had left Josephine's bed and had moved on to other ladies, I heard a shriek from Madeleine who still hovered over our comatose friend. *"Wendy! Tu as donne l'espoir! Venez ici immediatement!"* Yes, I had given hope but why the urgent call to return to Josephine? I quickly walked over to find that Josephine had awakened from the coma! Kneeling next to her, I saw the glazed, almost delirious, eye movement.

Josephine stared at me. There was a smile! There was a response to my touch. The family members were in disbelief. What had I done to release Josephine from the 'terminal coma'? The family cried, my colleagues cried, and I was totally weeping. Goose bumps. More tears, so touched, so encouraged, so deeply moved. Josephine gently squeezed my hand. Barely audible was the whisper, *"Ni nkupenda,"* Swahili for "I love you" from Josephine.

As I sat at the monastery that evening, I broke my solemn mood of the hospital, recalling how my arrival into Kinshasa, the capital of Congo-DRC, had been a total nightmare. After thirty-six hours of travel from Los Angeles, through Washington, DC, a six-hour layover in Paris, where I was so tired I just stared at nothing, I finally arrived to Kinshasa, three hours late.

The immigration area was a madhouse of Congolese scratching at my backpack to get my agreement for them to retrieve my luggage. Of course I had grabbed the baggage cart with stuck wheels. One bag. Finally, the second. Where was the suitcase with my clothes? It was lost. And where were my sponsors who had promised to meet me at immigration? The movement and circles of bags on the claim belt was nauseating. I finally accept the help of two rather scrappy looking fellows. I had the three huge duffels with training supplies for all three locations in the Congo: Brazzaville, Goma, Kinshasa.

As the last Air France passenger, I finally emerged from immigration, three hours after the plane landed. Twenty-five taxi drivers descended on me like flies to sticky paper. Where was that familiar handwritten sign *"Wendy,"* to connect me with the NGO sponsors? I explain in French that I am waiting for my friend. They try to convince me that 'my friend' told *them* to pick me up. I ask for the name of the man who was my supposed 'friend', and of course they have none. I think to myself, *"Didn't fool me this time, guys!"*

I paid one fellow $5 to borrow his cell phone to call Jean-Marie, who, I soon found, had apparently come to the airport and waited only thirty minutes, then assumed I had missed the flight and left. He was already back in Kinshasa but could return in ninety minutes. It was already 1:00 a.m., and I was ludicrous with fatigue and hunger.

Yes, I am truly back in Africa.

I return to the memories of the monastery where it is now after 10:00 p.m. Frickin' rat, resembling a football on feet, just ran over my sneakers. Now the bugs have crawled inside my dress and traverse unmentionable areas. I try to wrap another skirt around my legs to create a barrier to the flying things that commit suicide by flying into the candle flame. It smells like a bug BBQ of toasted wings and charred bodies. Of course I could just give up and go to bed, but this writing is therapeutic and I'm lost in the moment, so to speak.

I think I'm a bit homesick for the family.

Keeping On

Why are Michael's death and his last breath and the smell of the hospital room and the sounds as I walked down the corridor back to my car still so vivid, so real, so tangible to me? And why do I continue to fight for my stand of being controversial and being in a field where there is still so much discrimination and still so many stigmas?

One of my greatest frustrations is why I'm still giving the same information year after year after year—I'm saying the exact same thing now in 2012 that I was saying in 1982. That's thirty years. Thirty years we've known there are only three ways the virus goes from one person to another—we know exactly how to stop the virus. Yet when I started my work there were only 500 AIDS cases in the U.S., and now there are over 1.5 million!

Why is this happening in the United States, where we

have all this information, all this education, and the luxury of modern science, good teachers and transportation? I can see why I'm saying the same thing year after year after year in places like Africa and developing countries, because they simply have not had the information, they didn't know about AIDS. People were dying and they just thought that they were dying, but now we have a name for AIDS. But why here, in the U.S.?

And I have a lot of frustration with why we can't talk about prevention in specific religious communities. If we can't talk about condoms, we can't talk about AIDS prevention. Yet high school students quickly pull me aside and say, *I'm having sex, so what am I gonna do? How can I keep myself protected?*

And why is the government not doing more about this? I take all of these questions, and they fuel my drive, they fuel my passion to get in there and see if in this big rock I can't find some specks of gold. And there are some. Because just when you think everything is bad and exhausted, yet another slap in the face so you have to turn the cheek, then suddenly something positive appears.

I was in Kenya, in the slums of Mukuru, outside of Nairobi, walking in human excrement and animal feces and garbage, walking for about two kilometers in 112 degree temperature and slowly making my way to this mud hut, where I was invited to meet 150 Kenyans. I finally got there, and it turned out to be a very cramped 25 foot by 25 foot space, with absolutely no fresh air.

When this group of Kenyans saw Muzungu Wendy, they immediately thought, *Wow, a white person, we're gonna get some money from her, she's gonna help contribute to our community.* So one person was selected to talk about how there was no sanitation and no food and no electricity, and another person talked about the devastation of AIDS and the lack of information and everybody dying. They just went on and on and on about all of the problems in the community, and when it came time for me to talk, I just looked at them quite serenely and quite carefully and made eye contact with as many as possible.

Then with a bit of a smile on my face I asked, "How many of you can see Muzungu Wendy with your eyes, please raise your hand." They all raised their hands. I said, "How many of you can hear my voice?" They all raised their hands. "How many of you had something to eat today?" They all raised their hands, and I could see they were smiling. And I said, "Let's look at what we have, not what we don't have. So often we think we are the worst off, and then we see there's always something we have, there's always something we can do," and they all clapped.

So I do find the positive in so many of these very difficult situations, find there are some positive aspects to even HIV and AIDS. Yes, there's a tremendous amount of death and despair and frustration and sadness, but the people who are dying—and they know they're dying— share with me their deepest thoughts, their love of life, their sorrows, their hopes.

They've honestly taught me to stop and smell a rose. I appreciate the small things of life so much more now. If you don't just take all of this negativity and all this sadness, and instead put it together in a ball of momentum to keep persevering, there can be tremendous satisfaction, even when you reach just one person.

Working in 28 countries has been enthralling. There is so much homogeneity in spite of totally different cultures! And it's been a privilege to be a speaker with the U.S. State Department. They've sponsored HIV/AIDS prevention trainings in Namibia, Malawi, Zimbabwe and Ghana. It's such a treat for a change to have comfortable accommodations, per diems and a driver to shuttle us between events, with venues perfectly prepared and participants carefully selected. I feel so spoiled now that it might be a challenge to return to mud huts, goat intestines filled with stomach, outhouses, and exposure to myriads of insects.

I have a particular fondness for the continent of Africa. Having worked in thirteen African countries I have the highest respect for their culture, traditions and values. Their friendship and hospitality are genuine as they welcome me to their families and churches. They are receptive, hungry for information and motivated by the fact that they have lost too many friends and family members to HIV/AIDS.

I haven't traveled to Africa since my last assignment to Ghana with the US State Department. I was sidelined first

243

by a ripped-out quadriceps tendon complicated by serious hospital-induced infections, then by a total of eighteen knee surgeries which have kept me in a wheelchair for the past two years.

The hours and hours of waiting for improvements have stymied my ebullience and zapped my usual indefatigable energy. But it could be so much worse! Living with impoverished communities of HIV/AIDS-afflicted people has made me cherish what I have, more so than what I am missing.

In the end, though, it's still about choices. I choose every day. You have to. We all have choices—that's how we become who we are. I 'take the road less traveled'. I made choices—yes, I did! And I don't regret them. I've lived each day of my life in celebration, and my passions are *mine*. I've managed to follow them to make a difference in *my own way*. I wouldn't have it any other way. It's been *some* trip so far! And more choices still lie ahead!

PEP/LA International Programs

The Peer Education Program of Los Angeles (PEP/LA) is a non-profit organization in which multi-cultural teens from high schools, residential facilities and probation centers are trained to be peer educators in HIV/AIDS information. The mission of PEP/LA is two-fold: 1) to decrease the rising incidence of HIV transmission in adolescents; and 2) to elevate the care, respect, compassion and hope of people who live with HIV/AIDS.

PEP/LA has established 25 Peer Education Programs (PEPs) throughout Southern California, ("PEP/Satellites") the United States and has set up more than *120 teen* PEPs and *80 "Train the Trainers"* workshops in 28 countries *(PEP/INTERNATIONAL)*. Since 1986 most of these programs (listed below) continue to be successful in reaching teenagers with HIV/AIDS prevention. We look forward to welcoming several more African countries into our family of more than 12,600 teens and 8,800 "Trainers" who have been trained directly under the PEP/LA model.

Respecting cultural, ethnic and economic differences, PEP/LA has designed training agendas that are flexible and can be adapted to the specific concerns of each country. Innovative strategies for involving multi-disciplinary participants from political, academic and medical arenas have led to the development, implementation, evaluation and revision of international PEPs that effectively reach adolescents with vital life-saving messages about how to avoid an exposure to HIV and how to stop the discrimination of people who live with HIV/AIDS.

Our appreciation to the following governmental and non-governmental (NGOs) sponsors:

1. **PEP/ARMENIA** – (1998) – (Yerevan). Sponsors: Armenian Ministry of Health, Ministry of Education and Science and Scientific Association of Medical Students of Armenia (SAMSA).

2. **PEP/BELIZE** – (1997, 1998) – 5 PEPs (Belize City, Orange Walk, Punta Gorda, San Pedro,

Corozal). Sponsors: Pan American Health Organization (PAHO), UNICEF, UNAIDS, Belize National AIDS Task Force.

3. **PEP/CAMEROON** – (2003) – 2 PEPs. (Limbe, Magunje, Mutengene). Sponsors: Association for the Rehabilitation and Wellbeing of Youth (ARWY), Province Hospital of Limbe, Limbe Coffee Processing Company, Cameroon Baptist Convention, The German Cooperation (GPS), others.

4. **PEP/CONGO**-Brazzaville - (2006) 1 PEP. Sponsors: AZUR Development, Silvia Niombo.

5. **PEP/CONGO-DRC** - (2006) 3 PEPs (Kinshasa, Goma). Sponsors: "ILDI-ONGD", "Marman Lamukas", "MIDEFHOPS", Isidore Kalimira.

6. **PEP/GHANA** – (2003, 2004, 2010) – 9 PEPs. (Kumasi, Agona, Accra, Bipoah Ashanti, Patriensa, Buduburam, Elmina, Kissi). Sponsors: Rural Youth Development Association in Kumasi, Ashanti Health Services of the Ministry of Health, Asante-Akim Multipurpose Telecommunication Centre (AAMCT) of Patriensa, Mt. Olive Presbyterian

Church of Patasi, Self-Help Initiative for Sustainable Development (SHIFSD) of Buduburam, Komenda Edina Eguafo Abirem (KEEA) of Elmina District Council, Kingsby Hotel in Accra. In 2010: Embassy in Accra, West African AIDS Foundation (WAAF), Ghanian Military/

7. **PEP/GUYANA** - (1994) – (Nieuw-Nickerie). Sponsors: PAHO, Suriname National AIDS Programme.

8. **PEP/HUNGARY** - (1993, 1994, 1995) – 5 PEPs. (Budapest, Zalaegerszeg, Eger, Gyor, Heves County). Sponsors: Semmelwies University of Medicine, Swiss-Hungarian AIDS Prevention Effort (SHAPE), Hungarian Ministry of Social Welfare, City Councils of Zalaegerszeg, Eger, Gyor and Heves County, more.

9. **PEP/INDIA** – (2001) – 5 PEPs. (Nellore). Sponsors: Health, Education and Rural Training Society (HEARTS), Indian Ministry of Health and Social Welfare, Indian Red Cross of Hyderabad.

10. **PEP/ISRAEL** – (1992, 1995) – 2 PEPs. (Rishon-Le-Zion, Givatayim). Sponsors: Kupat Holim

Health Insurance, Israeli Association of Health Education.

11. **PEP/KENYA** – (2000, 2004) – 3 PEPs.. (Nakuru, Kiambu, Machakos). Sponsors: Learning and Development Kenya in Nakuru, Ark Foundation (Washington, DC), Uzima Wa Taifa (UZIWATA) in Kiambu, New Lifestyle Resource Centre of Machakos, District Women Council on HIV/AIDS (DIWOCHA), Development Services of the Catholic Diocese in Machakos.

12. **PEP/LA- USA** – Since 1990. Sponsors: Kaiser Permanente Hospital, Buffalo Club, Namaste Foundation, Entertainment Industries Foundation (EIF), California Endowment, Blue Cross Health Net, McDonnell Douglas Employee Fund, Edison, Ludacris Foundation, UCLA, Moorpark College, USC,.Buckley School, Oakwood School, Brentwood School, Macy's Passport West, individual donors, fundraisers.

13. **PEP/LIBERIA** - (2008) 6 PEPs (Monrovia) Sponsors: LOA, SHIFSD, Obaas School, YOCADS.

14. **PEP/MALAWI** - (2010) 4 PEPs. (Lilongwe, Blantyre, Salima) Sponsor: US Embassy in Lilongwe.

15. **PEP/MOSCOW** - (1991, 1992, 1993, 1994, 1995, 1996) – 7 PEPs. Sponsors: Moscow City Parliament, Moscow Duma, Russian Red Cross, AIDS-Infoshare Russia, AESOP, HERA, Prospeckt Mira.

16. **PEP/NAMIBIA** - (2006, 2010) 8 PEPs. (Windhoek, Rundu,Rehobeth, Grootfontein, Walvis Bay,Penduka) Sponsors: US Embassy in Windhoek, "Youth for Hope", Youth to Youth", American Cultural Center of the US Embassy.

17. **PEP/NANJING-China** – (1997) 2 PEPs. Sponsors: State Family Planning Commission of China, Nanjing College for Population and Programme Management (NCPPM).

18. **PEP/NEPAL** – (1996, 2001, 2005) – 4 PEPs. (Kathmandu) Sponsors: "Forum Against AIDS, Drugs and Social Problems" (FADS), Save the Children US-Kathmandu, National Federation of UNESCO Clubs in Nepal (NAFUCIN), UNESCO

International, Gandaki Seva Samaj Society, Chomolungma UNESCO Centre (CUC), Buddha UNESCO Club.

19. **PEP/PARIS**-France – L'Association "Jeunes" Contre le SIDA (L'AJCS), L'Association "Jeunes" Information contre le SIDA (L'AJIS) (1986, 1987, 1994, 1998) Sponsors: L'Association des Artistes Contre le SIDA (L'AACS), Mayor of Paris, Fondation Recherche Medicale, French Ministry of Health.

20. **PEP/PHILIPPINES** – (1996) – 2 PEPs.. (Cebu City) Sponsors: Bidisliw Foundation in Cebu City, Save the Children US – Cebu.

21. **PEP/PUERTO RICO** – (1992) 2 PEPs. (San Juan, La Perla) Sponsors: Harvard Institute for International Development, San Juan AIDS Institute.

22. **PEP/RUSSIA and PEP/SIBERIA** – (1992, 1996, 1997, 2000, 2003) 6 PEPs. (Omsk, Tomsk, Barnaul, Vladivostok) Sponsors: AIDS-Infoshare Russia, Omsk Regional AIDS Centre, Tomsk "Siberia AIDS Aid", Barnaul "Siberian Initiative",

UNICEF, Vladivostok Organization "LUBLU", Vladivostok Organization "LIFE".

23. **PEP/SOUTH AFRICA** – (2000, 2005) 5 PEPs. (Potchefstroom, Ikegeng, Dennilton, Houghton, Alexandra-Soweto) Sponsors: University of Natal - Durban, Nelson Mandela Medical School - Durban, Die Afrikanerbond – Johannesburg, Potchefstroom University School of Social Welfare, Rotary Club of Potchefstroom, NextAID, Youth with a Vision – Dennilton, Association Francois Xavier Bagnoud (AFXB)- Johannesburg.

24. **PEP/SURINAME** – (1993, 1994, 1996, 1997) 4 PEPs. (Paramaribo, Niew-Nickerie) Sponsors: Pan American Health Organization (PAHO), Suriname National AIDS Programme.

25. **PEP/TANZANIA** – (2005, 2007, 2008, 2010) 10 PEPs. (Dar es Salaam, Tanga, Boko, Mbeya, Chalinze, Mbalizi, Ituha, TEKO University, Kisanga) Sponsors: ARK AFRICA Foundation in Washington, DC Unity in Diversity (UDF) in Mbeya. In 2010: UDF Iringa Residential Training Foundation (IRTF), Mbalizi/Mbeya Presbyterian

Church, Malezi Alive Pioneers (MAP), MBeya Hope for Orphans (MBEHO).

26. **PEP/THAILAND** – (1995) 2 PEPs. (Bangkok) Sponsors: Chulalongkorn University of Medicine in Bangkok, Thai Red Cross.

27. **PEP/UGANDA** – (2000, 2002, 2005, 2007) 12 PEPs. (Kyebando, Kayunga, Kayonza, Galiraya, Busaana, Bukolooto, Namugongo, Mayuge, Jaguzi Island, Busuyi) Sponsors: FARE Ministries of Kampala, Kampala Baptist Union, Kayunga District Council, Youth and People with Disabilities Integrated Development Association (YOPDIDA), Uganda Health Empowerment Project (UHEP), Kayonza Council, Kon. Minister Rukia Isanga Nakadama (Ministry of Gender and Culture).

28. **PEP/ZIMBABWE** – (1999, 2010) 4 PEPs. (Magenje, Chivende, Harare, Bulawayo) Sponsors: Ministry of Health of Zimbabwe, Ivainesu Health Project of Karoi, Karoi Hospital. In 2010: US Embassy in Harare.

After arrival into a country, it takes about two weeks for the PEP/LA Trainer(s) to work with the hosting organizations for scheduling community forums, planning the training sessions for the teen peer educators, and conducting the *"TRAIN THE TRAINERS" Workshops* for 30-40 diverse participants (medical care professionals, school counselors, teachers, psychologists, Directors of NGOs, sex workers, family planning clinicians, rural health care workers, pastors, women's groups, prison staff, etc.). These "trainers" (more than 6,000 worldwide) then take the strategies of "peer education" to reach their respective populations with HIV/AIDS prevention and health promotion. The series of discussions focus on:

1. Negotiation and communication skills;
2. Recommendations for setting up their own PEP (for adults and/or teens);
3. Basic HIV/AIDS medical information to insure standardization of messages shared with targeted groups; and
4. Recommendations for counseling men, women and children living with HIV/AIDS.
5. The PEP/LA "Trainer(s)" help with the foundation

254

of the PEP onto which they will develop components that are culturally appropriate to their own country. Hence, the PEP is not a transplanted USA project; it will be successful only if they take full responsibility and ownership.

For the PEER EDUCATORS' TRAINING, the 50-55 adolescents (17-25 years old) are often recruited from medical schools, high schools, church groups and orphanages. In 3-4 days (a total of 18-24 hours), the teens participate in a series of informal discussions that cover:

1. Why teens are particularly at high risk;
2. The essentials of HIV/AIDS (*"AIDS 101"*);
3. Communication and public speaking skills;
4. "Cardinal rules" of confidentiality, empathy, honesty and non-judgmental attitudes. The trainees are empowered with decision-making skills, heightened self-esteem and positive health/ sexuality. The program information is transferable to the reduction of risk-taking behaviors of teens in general (drugs / alcohol / STDs / unwanted pregnancies). There is an emphasis on the goal of disease prevention through the promotion of

healthy life-styles. With community mobilization, the international PEP Directors then implement activities such as program promotion, peer educators' presentations, role-playing exercises and also provide HIV antibody testing information relevant to their own country's resources; and,

5. The provision of care compassion, hope and health care to people living with HIV/AIDS and their families.

On a worldwide scale, the PEP/LA satellite programs of PEP/INTERNATIONAL clearly improve HIV/AIDS knowledge and communication skills of youth and "Trainers". Pre/post-test questionnaires also document positive changes (26% + 7%) in attitudes and intentions to modify risk behaviors associated with HIV transmission.

There is no doubt that the PEPs have also contributed to the understanding that discrimination against people with HIV/AIDS must be stopped and we must provide them with hope, care and medicines.

Author

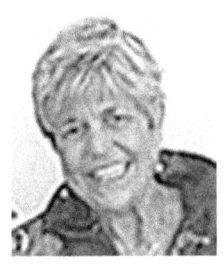

Wendy Arnold was brought up in Concord, Massachusetts and received her Masters Degree in Public Health from the Jonathan and Karin School of Public Health, UCLA, Los Angeles. She has passionately worked in HIV/AIDS education and care since 1982. With her international colleagues, Wendy has helped establish more than 180 Peer Education Programs (PEPs) in 28 countries. Africa has been her focus since 1999. Here in Los Angeles, Wendy is the Director of PEP/LA (www.pepla.org), where teens talk openly and directly with teens residing in out of school facilities, group homes, probation centers and runaway/homeless shelters. Annually, PEP/LA leads discussions with more than 4,000 youth and 500 adults who are therapists, case workers and counselors for these troubled teens. PEP/LA's educational outreach is highlighted with personal testimonies of our friends living with HIV/AIDS. Her three yellow Labradors keep her happy and busy in West LA.